Bad Stuff Out + Good Stuff in = Health

Your formula to being healthy in the modern world

Dr. Shania Seeber

Copyright © 2024

All rights reserved.

All rights reserved. No part of this publication may be reproduced, distributed, or transmitted in any form or by any means, including photocopying, recording, or other electronic or mechanical methods, without the author's prior written permission, except in the case of brief quotations embodied in critical reviews and certain other non-commercial uses permitted by copyright law. For permission requests, please get in touch with the author.

Contents

Dedication i
Acknowledgment ii
About the Author iii
Introduction 1
Chapter 1: What is the Bad Stuff 7
Chapter 2: How Do These Bad Things Cause Damage 16
Chapter 3: A Brief Introduction on How to Assess the Bad Stuff 19
Chapter 4: What is the Good Stuff 24
Chapter 5: What Does It Feel Like to Heal 38
Chapter 6: Prepping for Detoxification and Covering the Bases 43
Chapter 7: Important Vitamins and Co-Factors 51
Chapter 8: Diving Deeper into Detoxification & Dealing with The Bad Stuff 55
Chapter 9: The Basics of Genes and Enzymes 74
Chapter 10: Methylation Genes 77
Chapter 11: Detoxification Genes 81
Chapter 12: Inflammation Genes 83
Chapter 13: Oxidative Stress Genes 85
Chapter 14: Genes That Infer a Higher Need for Certain Nutrients 88
Chapter 15: Heavy Metals and Why They Are Bad 92
Chapter 16: Testing for Heavy Metals 99
Chapter 17: Mould 112
Chapter 18: Managing Moisture to Prevent Mould Growth 123
Chapter 19: Mycotoxins 127
Chapter 20: Volatile Organic Compounds 133
Chapter 21: Plastics and Persistent Organic Pollutants 135
Chapter 22: Toxic People 139
Chapter 23: Still Got Chemical Sensitivities? 143
Chapter 24: Hormones - How They Are Affected by Bad Stuff 145
Chapter 25: A Guide to Using Food as Medicine 152
Chapter 26: Track and Reset Yourself 169
Chapter 27 – Reference Section for Toxic and Essential Elements 180
Chapter 28 - Reference Section for Mould Species 287
Chapter 29 - Reference Sections for The Specific Mycotoxins 297

Dedication

I would like to dedicate this book to my loving husband, John, who was like medicine while I was on my healing journey and is my constant support.

Acknowledgment

I would like to acknowledge my life experiences, without which I would never have grown the knowledge base I now have to share with you.

I would also like to acknowledge my teachers, in whatever form they chose to be, my family, my lecturers at university, my educators from The Institute of Functional Medicine Institute, my colleagues and friends in the industry and my patients, who have helped guide me through their experiences.

My illustrators, Nadine & Dominic, my website developer and friend, Richard and my proof-reading team, thank you!

I would also like to acknowledge whatever it was that guided you to pick up this book. It is a tool you can use to improve your health and I hope you gain what you need from it.

About the Author

Shania Seeber was born in a small mining town west of Johannesburg, South Africa. Her journey to figuring out her own root cause of health started at an early age and developed into a career in complementary alternative medicine.

She relocated to the United Kingdom in 2016 and has continued to guide patients and educate doctors in the UK on lifestyle medicine and root cause treatment, helping them to understand that the body can indeed heal itself, if you make sure the good stuff outweighs the bad stuff.

In this book, she offers her personal, practical insights on how to get the bad stuff (heavy metals, mould, persistent organic pollutants, and toxic relationships) out and get the good stuff (nutrients, positive thoughts & actions) in, so that your body can heal itself the way it is designed to.

She has written this as a guide for you. It is your formula for being healthy in the modern world.

Introduction

I firmly believe that I have gone through the life experiences I have had so that I can make the world a better place by making the people on it, better and healthier versions of themselves. Something must have drawn you to this book, so I hope the information in it can also help you heal from whatever is weighing you down.

That may sound dramatic, but, if it wasn't for the extreme exposure to heavy metals and mould that I experienced firsthand, I wouldn't know what I know about them. I was not taught about them at university, so, when I got sick, I was forced to search for and learn about solutions to get better. Most importantly, if I hadn't gone through all of this, I wouldn't be sharing these experiences and this knowledge with you!

I was already a qualified doctor of complementary alternative medicine when I realised, I was seriously chronically sick and not getting the answers I needed from my university training. To give you some perspective, I had 5 years of full-time university training and a year of supervised clinic work under my belt, when I suffered not my first, but my most severe, episode of chronic fatigue and fibromyalgia (chronic pain syndrome).

Let me go back a few years to the first episode.

At age 7, I was my school's youngest ever champion swimmer. I was a natural, and I won the following year too. Things were looking good for me. Until one day, at aged 9, I woke up with swollen glands in my neck and armpits and couldn't even lift my arms from the severe fatigue. I was misdiagnosed with mumps because my glands were swollen and sore. Over the next few months, I was prescribed numerous courses of antibiotics, which had no effect on the symptoms and completely wrecked my poor guts! Six months later, someone recommended a Naturopath to my now desperate mother. I remember that consultation well, the man who asked so many questions and did a more thorough investigation than any of the other doctors before him. I don't know what he gave me but 2 weeks later, 6 months after I fell "ill," I was better, and I had my energy back. But I wasn't cured, because sadly, a few years later, the symptoms came back!

The next episode that remains in my memory was when I was 17, in my final year of school and part of the A team of our school for hockey. Life was generally good until one day, I woke up, and the short walk to the kitchen felt like I had run a marathon, it was exhausting. I was also in pain, so much pain. This was my first experience of fatigue with fibromyalgia or chronic pain syndrome. Everything hurt, and it wasn't easy to do anything. I went from being on the A team, to being on the bench and feeling like I was on the brink of death. This was diagnosed as another viral infection and also stuck around for about 6 months.

In my 3rd year of university, I had my next episode. This was longer and way more severe. Along with the fatigue and pain came a mental darkness I can only describe as having my soul sucked out of my body. I had no more of the light I knew myself to have; the happiness and joy I was known for was gone. The vibrant, energetic and fun person people knew me to be, was gone. For almost a year, I am sad to say; I wanted to die. I went to various doctors and even to a psychiatrist, but all my tests came back normal, and the medications prescribed for the depression only made me worse, and eventually, I was told that all the pain, the darkness, and suffering was 'in my head.' In a last-ditch attempt to heal myself, I visited the student clinic at my university, and 2 young students took my case and convinced me to "hang in there" while they worked out my remedy. I returned a week later, and they gave me a remedy. Within a few moments, I started to feel different, and an hour later, I felt almost euphoric. This euphoria was not drug-induced. It was my light, my joy, my usual self, returning. I was cured... for a short while at least.

The last serious and by far the worst episode of fatigue and pain began when I was 28 years of age, and by now, I was a competitive mountain biker. I was recently married, and we were moving across the country. Life should have been perfect. My young husband left 2 months before me to find work and a home. During these 2 months, things went horribly wrong with my health. I was more exhausted than in any of the previous episodes. I gained weight, and I lost my light again. My new husband, not knowing what had happened, had bought us mountain bikes to enjoy riding around Cape Town, but I rode about 100m and threw up. I couldn't recover from the exhaustion of that short ride. Something was seriously wrong, and I needed to know what.

I was now desperate and went to any doctor I could to get to, both conventional and naturopathic. I did every test available by general doctors and even naturopaths. However, all the tests I did came back "normal" again. It took me 6 years, and many doctors telling me my pain and severe fatigue was "all in my head" to find MY "root cause." In this case, it was massive amounts of heavy metals!

To explain why I had these heavy metals, I need to explain where I was exposed. The town I was born in and lived in for the first 13 years of my life, was a mining town. It was literally a mine dump. A mine dump is where the minerals and metals that aren't gold or something "useful" are dumped as mountains of fine dust around the area. This dust then blows into the air, and we breathe it, eat it, and drink it. I also had an awful dentist who gave me mercury fillings at every visit. His nickname was Bill, due the fact that regardless of the health of your teeth, when you went to see him, he would drill, fill and bill. This only compounded my personal exposure to heavy metals like mercury.

Now, I must make it clear, exposure to the occasional metal is not a bad thing for everyone. Some people get sick, and others don't. Or they get entirely different symptoms! It depends on how much they were exposed to, how long they were exposed and other fun things like genetics. In my family, my brother had severe eczema but never had crippling fatigue; my mom had chronic sinus issues. My father occasionally had gout, which I now know can be caused by oxidative stress increasing uric acid! I guess my point it that we all had the same exposure but presented with different symptoms. This is why toxins can confuse the average medical professional!

In 2008, I went to a functional medicine conference and discovered that along with the vast exposure to heavy metals, I also don't have genetically optimally functioning enzymes for removing heavy metals. So, the massive exposure to the heavy metals compounded by the non-functioning enzymes that are needed to remove them meant an added body burden over time. I don't have terrible genes, but both methylation and glutathione conjugation of heavy metals (the 2 main ways you remove heavy metals from your body) are compromised and need loads of support in the form of toxin avoidance and specific nutrition.

My next step was to learn how to remove heavy metals from my body, which I did successfully, and life should have been amazing, right?

On 1st December 2012 (I was now a much healthier version of myself), I moved into a new house. I could smell "damp," but I didn't think anything of it. On the 25th of December, I had my first-ever nosebleed. It was random. I was in my late 30s and never had a nosebleed. Well, I had many after that! Almost daily! I later discovered this is one of the many symptoms caused by mould toxicity! Welcome to my next "Bad Thing!"

I then developed so many more symptoms that I won't list here; you can read about them in the chapter on mould.

With this vast personal experience of these 2 major environmental toxins, I made them one of the main focuses of my practice. I learned quickly that most people with chronic fatigue, pain, immune or hormonal conditions have some kind of toxic burden, which means hormones and enzymes don't function optimally. The good news is, that I also found that the body is amazing at healing itself when you take the bad stuff out and put the good stuff back in.

Over time, through working with both my own patients and then with practitioners moving into functional or lifestyle medicine, I noticed a trend to overcomplicate the underlying root causes and treat the body as if all symptoms were caused by a linear process of insult to injury. This is, unfortunately, not a helpful way to think about health or healing.

The fact is that simplifying the approach to understanding healing is often more helpful to both the patient and the practitioner. Take the bad stuff out, put the good stuff in... and you will heal!

A "less is more" approach is also better when working with someone who has multiple symptoms with multiple causes. I like to describe the process as more of a "spider web" where even the most minor action can be significant and sometimes just focusing on the top priorities will get you spontaneous results in other areas. The way I explain this is if you have a spider in a web and you want to get its attention, you stimulate the web in 1 or 2 maybe 3 close areas, not every region around the web! That would confuse the spider, and most likely freak it out, whereas stimulating just one small area, the spider would focus on that area, would move to it, and repair it!

Although most people want to, I don't encourage people to do an "everything all at once" approach as it seldom works and can make them worse. Focus on the basics and the top 3 main issues you have and surprisingly enough, you will find they will be resolved, and you can then focus on the next set of issues. Healing is a journey and has many layers and adaptations on the way, so don't do what everyone who is sick wants to do and try to fix everything all at once, because that doesn't work, you will be as overwhelmed as a spider with too many flies in its web.

Hopefully, this book will clear your path, reveal YOUR top 3 priorities, and assist you on your journey.

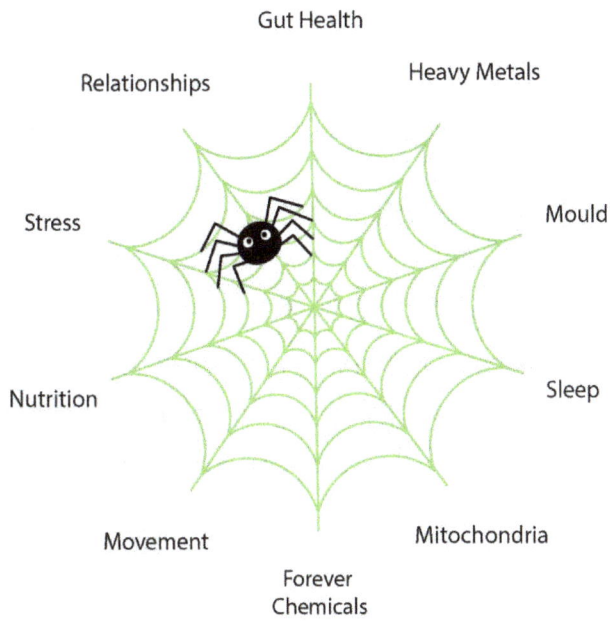

The spider web approach of helping the body to heal: Everything is connected. If you focus on the top 2-3 areas of concern and address those, then the next layers will surface and can be addressed. Sometimes they even resolve themselves because the other issues were dealt with. Here the spider is working on stress, relationships and gut health, leaving the rest for now!

Something we sadly seem to have forgotten over time, is that our body is built to heal. If we feed it the "Good Stuff" and avoid and remove as much of the "Bad stuff", it will naturally move to a more energised, pain-free, healthier self! I am glad to say I am living proof of this fact!

This is why I am grateful for the exposures I have had and the experience they gave me. Without having gone through the experience myself, I would never have known that you can indeed be energetic, pain-free, and happy even with a history of chronic fatigue, pain, and depression... there is a light at the end of the tunnel that I can now share with you!

The role of this book is to simplify what can become an overly complicated topic and to arm you with all the tools you need to process whatever is currently burdening you to get you on track for recovery. There are many good books on the topics discussed in this book that go much deeper into the science, and I encourage you to read more.

I must add that I am not a fan of "protocols," so I will give general guidelines and tools both in this book and on my website, but you need to follow what works for you! I also highly recommend working with someone with experience in the field who can be objective about your experiences, even if you are a healthcare practitioner! You need someone else to have an objective view of your symptoms.

For those wondering whether there have been any recurrence of depression, pain or fatigue, thankfully I can say with confidence, that I have not had any an episode of anything chronic since around 2010. Still going strong!

Finally, my hope for you, if you are reading this because you, or someone you love is chronically ill, is that the tools provided to you in this book, make your life better!

Please use the companion information available on wwww.drshania.com along with the information in this book.

Chapter 1: What is the Bad Stuff

If you had asked me what I wanted to be when I grew up, when I was about 10 years old, my answer would have been, "a detective". I loved solving the crimes in the detective books that I had, so much so that as a young teenager, my answer had morphed to "a forensic scientist". It was only in my later teens, where I realized that I didn't really like the idea of working with gruesome crimes and that maybe there were other sorts of crimes I could solve. So that's how I decided to study how to heal people, rather than solve their cause of death. To me, symptoms are like clues at a crime scene and you, the sick person, are the crime scene and I now need to find the criminal. Every sick person's body is supplying evidence to the crime that is the root cause of their dis-ease. These are the symptoms and the test results, which are then used to discover who, or in this case, what, the criminal is. We can then address this and solve the crime so that the body can heal.

The criminals are the "Bad Stuff" that harm us. This bad stuff is often common, yet potentially toxic substances or actions that we are now exposed to more regularly than our ancestors were. These things can all negatively impact health to some degree, depending on factors such as how much you were exposed to and how long you were exposed to it for as well as factors like your genetics, lifestyle, and your nutrition status. We all get exposed to them these days, there is no escaping that, but we can learn to reduce the exposure and support our body's ability to remove them.

The bad stuff affects the way the body functions, and if they are substances we are exposed to (rather than bad habits or toxic relationships), they are usually fairly quickly removed from the body via the liver, kidneys, bowels, lungs, and skin. However, these organs and systems can be overwhelmed by the sheer amount they have to deal with on a daily basis, especially if we have excessive exposure or have genetically weak enzymes like I have, which are sadly very common.

Other "toxins," such as a sedentary lifestyle, bad sleep, stress, and toxic relationships, require a lifestyle change to be "detoxed," and this means some effort from you! Remember, you don't have to fix all of them at once, remember the spider in its web, work on the top priorities and once those are mastered, move onto the next.

Although there are many other substances that are considered toxic, such as some viruses and bacteria, EMFs (electromagnetic fields) or a toxin that is a poison produced naturally by an organism (e.g., plant, animal, insect.) for the purposes of this book, the "Bad stuff" will fall into one of the following categories:

Heavy Metals	Persistent Pollutants/Forever chemicals
Mould and the toxins they produce	Lifestyle and Relationships

It may seem strange that I have decided not to include pathogens like viruses and bacterial infections. The reason I chose not to include them is that in my experience, unless it is an acute infection that requires immediate treatment, in chronic conditions, while viruses can be active and bacterial infections can linger, in most cases of chronic disease, if you remove one or all of the aforementioned bad things, the immune system can then face those infections, and you will heal naturally. While you are burdened with bad stuff, the immune system cannot fight infections, and so there are very often active infections in people who have a toxic burden! My advice is to try to clean up your external and internal environments, check if that helps you resolve the infection and if not, go to a doctor well versed in functional medicine for additional help.

We are much more susceptible to toxic burdens these days as we have only recently become exposed to most substances that affect us, and our environment is sadly becoming more toxic as the years pass by. Sorry kids, on the plus side, science is working hard to solve this dilemma.

Let me dive deeper into why we are being exposed more now than ever by discussing the timeline of when these environmental toxins first appeared in our history. Remember, that we have evolved over millennia, and our genes (which make our enzymes) are designed to keep us healthy in a world that existed 150+ years ago... we just aren't prepared for the ever-increasing toxic load we are being exposed to these days!

In the timeline of our natural exposure to toxicants, mould would be the one we have been exposed to the longest. In fact, it is so tenacious and ubiquitous that it is referenced in the bible, and Nasa has stated that when the first settlers travel to Mars, mould might be one of the first things that may impact their health and survival. They found that black mould fungus can temporarily survive on Mars's tough terrain. Maybe someone should tell all those billionaires who are trying to relocate there.

As for our exposure to heavy metals, the earliest known mine for a specific mineral is coal from Southern Africa, from around 40,000 to 20,000 years ago. But mining did not become a significant industry until more advanced civilisations developed 10,000 to 7,000 years ago. The problem with mines is that ore mills generate large amounts of waste, called tailings. For example, 99 tons of waste is generated per ton of copper, with even higher ratios in gold mining – because only 5.3 g of gold is extracted per ton of ore, a ton of gold produces 200,000 tons of tailings. That's crazy. What's worse is that these tailings can be full of discarded toxic heavy metals like cadmium and lead.

Tailings are mostly dumped into ponds made from naturally existing valleys. Sadly, this now makes that water a dangerous source of toxic chemicals, such as heavy metals, sulphides and even radioactive content.

Thankfully, not every exposure to bad stuff like heavy metals, will cause a problem by being overtly toxic, but what happens is that due to exposure over time, the body becomes progressively more burdened by the stored toxins it hasn't been able to remove. This is termed total body burden.

Imagine your body is in a glass being filled with the bad things that can harm us. The liver, kidneys, skin and guts are holes in the glass that prevent the liquid from filling all the way to the top. Over time, everyday exposures can add up, causing the glass to overflow. When this happens, symptoms ranging from brain fog, pain, fatigue, skin conditions, asthma, allergies, and others can occur. They initially may seem like minor health concerns but, left unaddressed, can become more serious conditions.

Of these conditions, the most common are chronic fatigue and pain syndromes, autoimmune conditions, cardiovascular disease, neuropathies (nerve pain), endocrine disruption (by hormone disruptors), infertility, and a weakened immune system to name a few.

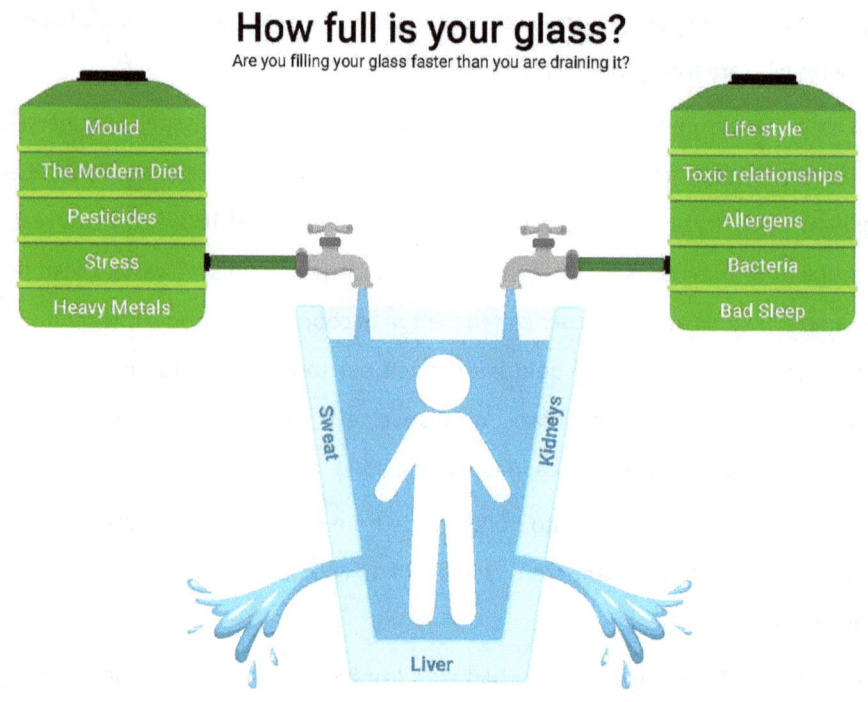

How full is your glass?

Persistent organic pollutants (also referred to as POP's or forever chemicals) have only been around since about the mid 1800's, when Eduard Simon, a German apothecary, discovered polystyrene. In 1856, a substance called Parkesine, the first member of the celluloid class of compounds and considered the first man-made plastic, was patented by Alexander Parkes.

Bisphenol A (BPA), a toxicant from plastic, known to be a major endocrine disruptor, which means it affects hormones, specifically oestrogen, was created by Thomas Zincke in 1966 at the University of Marburg, Germany. Later, a British chemist named Charles Edward Dodds was the first to recognise BPA as an artificial oestrogen and plastics were then required to be labelled BPA free. Sadly, the BPA free plastic options are not much better.

Another contributing factor (and a "bad thing") to our steadily declining health is our change in lifestyle over the past 100 years, from being active to being sedentary. From sleeping from sunset to dawn to being awake at all hours thanks to artificial light and the internet. From eating locally sourced foods to eating food marketed to us by the food industry. We now eat more heavily processed foods that contain more salt and sugar than our grandparents were ever exposed to. We have gone from eating nose to tail to eating fake meats. We ship our "fresh" food halfway around the world instead of keeping food local to the people who live in that area. Being mindful of where your food comes from is as important as eating for the nutritional value of that food!

The good news is that we can take back our power to heal. We can overpower the bad stuff with good stuff. We can also use certain foods to help remove environmental toxins. Foods such as good quality protein, organic or washed, locally sources, seasonal and colourful vegetables, and good quality fats from nuts, seeds, olives, and avocados can all help. Choosing to help your body with good food choices rather than harm it with bad ones is 1 step in the process of being a healthier version of yourself!

Sleep, exercise, and stress are all contributing factors to the spiderweb that creates health, and each one will need to be addressed and improved, along with removing any "bad stuff" and replacing it with the GOOD stuff!

The main sources of exposure to most bad things are:

Home, work, and cars:

We spend most of our lives in one of these 3 environments. Mould grows in most environments but is usually found in buildings that have even minor water damage, these buildings could be your home, a building you visit regularly, a musty hotel room etc. Another very common source of exposure to mould is cars! From air conditioning, spilled drink, windows left open in the rain etc. Most people can't see the mould and don't even know it is there. Sometimes the mould isn't even in or on their house or car, but a neighbour has mould that can affect the neighbourhood! The best thing to do is dehumidify and purify your air where possible. You can ozone your vehicle and home and get "fog" treatments done on your home that can help, but please, find the source of the damp and fix that before fogging. If you suspect mould is an issue, always treat the environment before attempting to treat yourself! Then there is the way we cook our food. Aluminium and copper cookware can leach those metals into acid food like tomatoes. Old buildings can have Lead (Pb) in the old paint. Microwaving or storing food in plastic can expose you to BPA and other plastic forever chemicals. Your cleaning and beauty products are yet another home source of bad things!

Air & water:

So, you can't really avoid air and water and I don't recommend you try, but you can filter both! Heavy metals like lead, mercury, cadmium, and arsenic often leach into drinking water and can accumulate in the body over time and cause various health problems. Lead exposure, especially in children, has been linked to developmental delays, decreased IQ, and behavioural issues. The most common sources of lead include breathing paint or dust, drinking water, using cosmetics that have them as ingredients, and some hobbies or jobs that include exposure to lead through air and skin.

Exposure to air pollutants that contain pollutants or even heavy metals, can lead to acute lung issues like asthma, bronchitis, and other lung diseases. Long-term exposure to air pollution is also associated with chronic conditions, including cardiovascular problems, chronic fatigue, brain fog, unexplained chronic pain, and increased mortality rates. The fact is that some people have no choice but to live in an area that has "bad air". Also, these particulates can travel halfway across the world unseen and unnoticed, which is why I always recommend good quality air purifiers in the bedroom, office and living room to ensure even the invisible particles won't affect you. Breathing clean air is essential!

Although tap water is generally considered safe in most first world countries, I still recommend filtering it as the levels of chlorine, copper and lead may vary depending on where you are. Contamination of drinking water sources with toxins like heavy metals (e.g., copper, lead, mercury, arsenic), pesticides, industrial chemicals, and microbial contaminants can cause a range of health problems. I recommend that people purify both the water they drink AND the water they shower or bath in if possible. Water purifiers come in all shapes, sizes and costs. My advice is to get something rather than nothing, because removing SOME of the bad stuff is better than removing none! Bottled water is fine if it is in glass or steel because water stored in plastic is a source of BPA and should be avoided wherever possible. If it's a choice between bottled water and dehydration, then by all means, please choose the bottled water and then support your detox pathways later.

Food:

Certain foods are more susceptible to leaching heavy metals, growing mould or being contaminated with forever chemicals. Acidic food cooked in certain metals will leach those metals into the food. Nuts, seeds and grain are often sources of exposure to mould. Left over foods are also prone to mould. Vegetables can be a source of bad herbicides and pesticides. To reduce your exposure, choose fresh, local ingredients and don't eat leftovers.

Prolonged or high-level exposure to some pesticides and herbicides has been linked to neurological disorders, hormone disruption, reproductive issues, and an increased risk of certain cancers. These chemicals don't break down easily and can be extremely difficult for the body to remove hence why they are called "persistent" or "forever" chemicals. To limit your exposure to them is to eat fresh, locally sourced, seasonal organic or washed fruit and veg.

You can always reference the dirty dozen (those fruit and vegetables that have the highest risk of being contaminated) and the clean fifteen (those fruit and vegetables that don't need to be "organic") online. This is a list of foods, updated annually by the Environmental Working Group (EWG) that tells you which fruit and vegetables need to be certified organic and which ones you can eat freely. The list does change every year or so, so keep an eye on them. Even better, grow your own fruit and vegetables.

As I mentioned, cookware used to prepare foods may also contribute to toxic metal exposure, especially if they were produced before the 1970s, so if you inherited pots and pans from your granny, please go and dispose of them now. Copper and aluminium cookware have been shown to leach toxic metals during cooking, especially when cooking with acidic foods like tomatoes.

The safest cookware materials include ceramic, glass, cast iron, and stainless steel. Using cast iron and stainless-steel cookware is generally considered safe, though, cooking with a cast iron pan may leach iron into foods, which is a potential benefit if individuals are deficient in this essential nutrient. However, excess iron may cause several health issues. Like cast iron, stainless steel may leach metals into foods, primarily nickel and chromium. Longer cook times above 20 hours, cooking acidic foods, and new or unused pots contributed to the most leaching. The best course of action is to avoid older products with contaminated glazes, cooking with acidic foods, and cleaning with abrasive sponges that may cause the release of unwanted bad things.

Other sources:

Other common sources of bad stuff are the cosmetics and cleaning agents we use daily. Exposure to potentially harmful chemicals found in everyday products, such as cleaning agents, pesticides, cosmetics, and plastics, can have adverse effects on our health over time. Please assess your cleaning products, use natural ones where possible, and remember that if you don't want to eat an ingredient in a product, you probably don't want to put it on your skin! Your skin absorbs all the bad things from cosmetics and beauty products in almost the same way as if you swallowed it.

It's important to note that the severity of the health effects caused by the "bad stuff" can vary depending on the level and duration of exposure, individual susceptibility, and other factors previously mentioned. Minimising exposure to environmental toxins using air purifiers and water purifiers, safe handling and disposal of chemicals, and adopting a healthy lifestyle can help reduce the impact that the bad stuff has on our bodies.

Even with the best habits in place, not all sources of exposure can be avoided. You can however; mitigate the effects by preventing toxic metals from being absorbed. Because many toxic metals and essential metals/minerals share similar sites of absorption, they may be taken up instead of the micronutrients needed by the body. What's more, essential micronutrient deficiencies may increase toxic metal absorption. For example, iron deficiency is associated with enhanced cadmium absorption. Similarly, a deficiency in calcium increases lead absorption. Therefore, the prevention of absorption, by having good nutrients in you, is imperative to avoid toxic metal uptake by the body.

These synergistic and antagonistic relationships are covered in the metals reference section of the book.

A note on stubborn weight and toxins

I know stubborn weight can be frustrating. As noted by the glass diagram, your body removes as many toxins as it can, as quickly as it can. Any that can't be processed and remain are stored, so that when the exposure is gone, the body can then safely remove those stored toxins. The unfortunate thing for most people is that fatty tissue is where most of the toxins are stored as a first line of storage, so the fat is there to protect you! People often notice a rapid increase in weight after an exposure to a toxicant. This is due to the body trying to dilute the toxin by retaining water. There is a saying in functional medicine that "the solution to pollution is dilution." This is also why many people report a quick loss of a few pounds/kilos in the Renew program, they are losing water, not fat. The fat loss comes later.

Stress is another bad thing that can also cause people to gain weight around the waist, so please manage your stress as part of any healthy weight loss journey!

Losing weight should be slow and done at the body's pace. If you lose that extra weight too fast and release too many stored toxins at once, you could make yourself sick. I've seen it in real life! Trust your body, that it knows what is best! You just make sure you have removed the bad stuff (toxins and stress) and are filling your glass with good stuff instead, so that you can heal!

Chapter 2: How Do These Bad Things Cause Damage

Symptoms created by a build-up of bad stuff over time, will occur when you reach your personal limit and you glass is now full of accumulated toxins that you weren't able to remove quickly or efficiently enough. In other words, your glass filled up faster than you can empty it and now you are overflowing with symptoms.

There are several ways that the bad stuff causes harm, but the main ways are through the oxidative stress and inflammation they create in us, along with suppressing many enzymes, interfering with hormones, messing with our energy makers (mitochondria) and microbiome. Basically, just impeding our normal functions through any means possible.

Let's start by looking at oxidative stress. You've seen oxidation in action in the form of rust, where iron has turned that distinct orange colour and isn't as strong as it used to be. Rust can literally break cars, so imagine what oxidative stress can do to you!

Oxidative stress is a condition that occurs when there is an imbalance between the reactive oxygen species (ROS), also known as free radicals, and the body's ability to neutralise them with antioxidants.

ROS's are highly reactive molecules that contain oxygen atoms with unpaired electrons. These electrons need to bind to something (an antioxidant) or else they bind to you, and they cause harm. They are produced as by-products of normal cellular processes, such as metabolism, and can also be created in response to external factors like pollution, radiation, and certain chemicals. Mould, mycotoxins, POP's, and heavy metals are all extremely oxidative and can create an excess of reactive molecules. These reactive molecules basically cause us to "rust" inside, just like you see rust on metal when it is left outside to oxidise!

Antioxidants are molecules that help neutralise ROS and prevent them from causing damage. They can be produced by the body, or you can get them from dietary sources, such as fruits, vegetables, and certain nutrients like glutathione and vitamins A, C, and E. When there is an excess of ROS or a deficiency of antioxidants, an imbalance occurs, leading to oxidative stress and dis-ease. ROS can react with and damage various cellular components, including lipids (fats), proteins, DNA, and cell membranes. This damage can disrupt normal cellular function and contribute to the development of various diseases and conditions.

Oxidative stress has been implicated in the development of chronic diseases, including cardiovascular disease, diabetes, neurodegenerative disorders, and cancer. It can contribute to tissue damage and accelerate the ageing processes. However, it's important to note that oxidative stress is a complex process influenced by various factors, and its role in disease development is still being studied. It is known, though, that oxidative stress can drive chronic inflammation. Let's discuss that next.

Inflammation is simply your immune system's response to an irritant. Whether that is an infection such as a cold virus or an injury such as a sprained ankle, and just about everything in between, including mould, heavy metals POP's and stress! If you're enjoying some sunshine on the deck with your family and get a splinter in your foot, you may notice the area around the splinter gets red and swollen. Or when you have the flu, you typically develop a fever as your body tries to kill the virus. Both these instances are examples of acute inflammation at work in your body, your inflammatory cells jumping in to fight against a potentially harmful injury or invader. This is a good thing. Unfortunately, if the response goes on longer than it should, the good, acute inflammation becomes bad, in that it is now chronic and needs to be shut down.

To mitigate oxidative stress and inflammation caused by heavy metals, moulds, and pollutants, it is important to maintain a healthy lifestyle that includes a balanced diet rich in protein and food-based antioxidants, regular physical activity, stress management, 7-8 hours of refreshing sleep, and avoidance of harmful environmental factors. There are foods and supplements that are also known to help reduce oxidative stress and inflammation. I'll go into detail about those later in the book.

Symptoms related to chronic exposure to environmental pollutants include:

Allergies	Headaches
Behaviour & mood disorders	Hormonal imbalances
Brain fog	Infertility in men and women
Cancer	Irritable bowel syndrome
Cardiovascular issues	Nose bleeds

Chronic fatigue	Obesity or Weight issues in general
Cognitive difficulties	PMS and extreme menopause symptoms
Degenerative neurological conditions	Skin conditions (eczema, psoriasis)
Fibromyalgia	And more

Basically, anything associated with modern-day chronic health problems.

Remember that not every exposure to a bad thing will cause a problem by causing immediate damage, but what happens is due to exposure over time, the body becomes progressively more burdened by the stored toxins it hasn't been able to remove. It is the glass being too full that creates the symptoms.

Chapter 3: A Brief Introduction on How to Assess the Bad Stuff

How do you know which bad thing you have been exposed to and now need to address? Maybe you only need to address heavy metals or mould, but these days, I am personally finding that patients often have many layers of things and need to address mould, heavy metals, pollutants, and more, all in a single case! But remember, don't address everything all at once, or you will overwhelm the spider in its web. Prioritise what needs to be addressed and work with the top 3 issues first.

There are specific tests that can help you to assess your total toxic burden and guide your program. There are details on the tests in their relevant chapters and I have a list of labs you can use at the back of the book. I won't mention any labs by name in the book though, because if you consult with a qualified professional, who knows how to runs lab tests, they may use a different yet equally relevant laboratory test. Also, new tests are being developed all the time, so some new tests may not be explicitly mentioned.

A fact about testing for any environmental toxin, that very few labs will admit to, is that they are all screening tests, not diagnostic, so that means they all have their pros and cons. None are 100% reproducible, none is "the best", BUT most will do well for screening and monitoring purposes. Remember that if the body is exposed to more than it can deal with in that moment, it will store it away to deal with it later. Aluminium and mercury are often stored in nervous tissue like the brain. If you really wanted to assess how much aluminium or mercury is in the brain, you would have to get a sample of brain tissue and analyse that. That's not possible or advisable. The best you can do, is get an idea of what the body has been exposed to and how it is potentially eliminating or storing it and work from there.

I also don't recommend attempting to actively remove any bad stuff until you are sure your gut bugs are happy and healthy. We are in essence, very complicated doughnuts, with a long doughnut hole going all the way through is. I will refer to it as "the tube." To assess the health of the tube and the bugs that live in it, we must assess the stuff that comes through the tube and out of it as waste. Yup, that means a poop test! I need to make it clear that poop tests are also NOT diagnostic tests, unless you are looking for something specific. They are screening tests that assess the overall health of your guts. Very few bacteria in themselves can influence your health unless they are pathogenic (disease causing), but the balance of the bugs can tell us whether the overall microbiome is healthy or not. We assess the patterns of dysbiosis. The most common pattern we see is caused by stress, not chewing and not having adequate stomach acid or digestive juices in general, to digest properly. When you are stressed, your body doesn't produce enough acid in your stomach which means that any bacteria on your skin or in your mouth (that live there naturally), can pass through the stomach, where the acid would normally obliterate them, and into the rest of your guts. If some of those bacteria end up in the colon, they can trigger all sorts of bad things, including inflammation in the gut, or worse, auto immunity or even cancer.

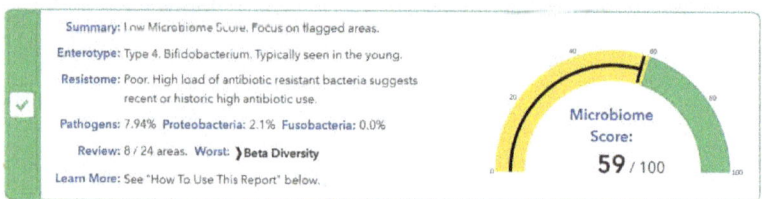

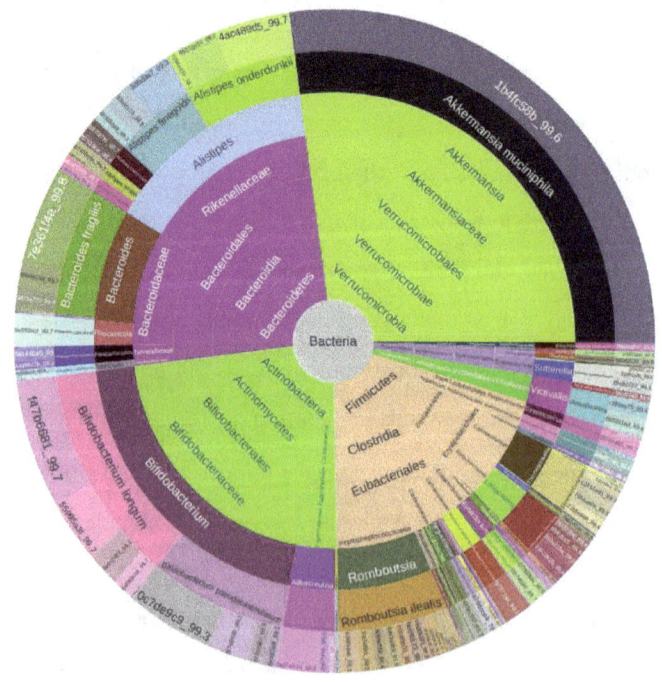

Here is just one example of a microbiome analysis report, isn't it pretty!

In this case we can see the pattern of markers in the test result shown in the diagram. This person needs to improve their microbiome diversity a little, they can do that by choosing better food and chewing it well so that the stomach can digest it better and the fibre can feed the good gut bugs and of course, working on their stress!

When testing for mould and mycotoxins, my personal approach involves using a urine test to evaluate mycotoxins along with organic acids (the end products of metabolism). If the patient I am working with also has issues with histamine and potential mast cell activation, then I include a blood test that looks at the IGE (an immunoglobulin that means you have an allergy and will get itchy and red symptoms on contact with that mould species), IGG (an immunoglobulin that can also mean you have an allergy but is more for confirming past exposure to certain moulds) and IGA (an immunoglobulin that can reveal current immunological activity to a certain mould, so you know what is in your current environment). Again, there are a few companies offering tests, so if your provider chooses another lab to the ones mentioned at the back of the book, that's OK!

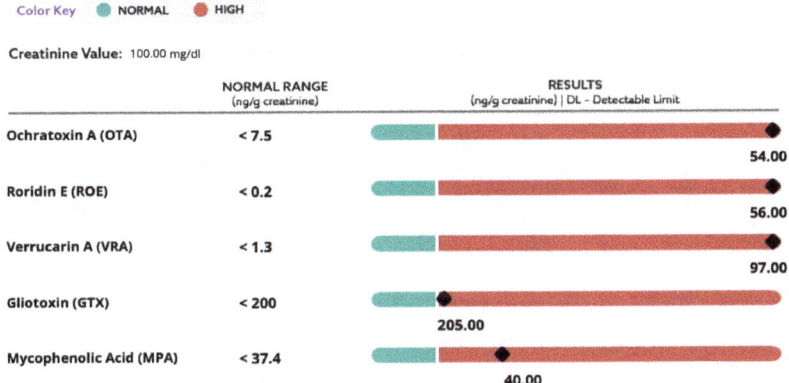

This is what a positive result for mycotoxins looks like from 1 specific lab, any black dot in the red part is BAD!

To screen for heavy metals, you can use hair, blood, urine and stool to assess past and current exposures or the body's detoxification of them. You won't be able to determine the exact load on any tissue without taking a piece of that tissue and examining that, and that would be incredibly invasive, so we work with what we have access to deduce the overall burden. I often use a combination of hair, blood and urine to assess for metals.

What is useful about hair is that it is relatively inexpensive, and it is also an accessible biopsy material that conveniently grows out of the body. Taking a sample generally causes very little trauma to the patient and gives an average over time of exposure and detoxification of the metals.

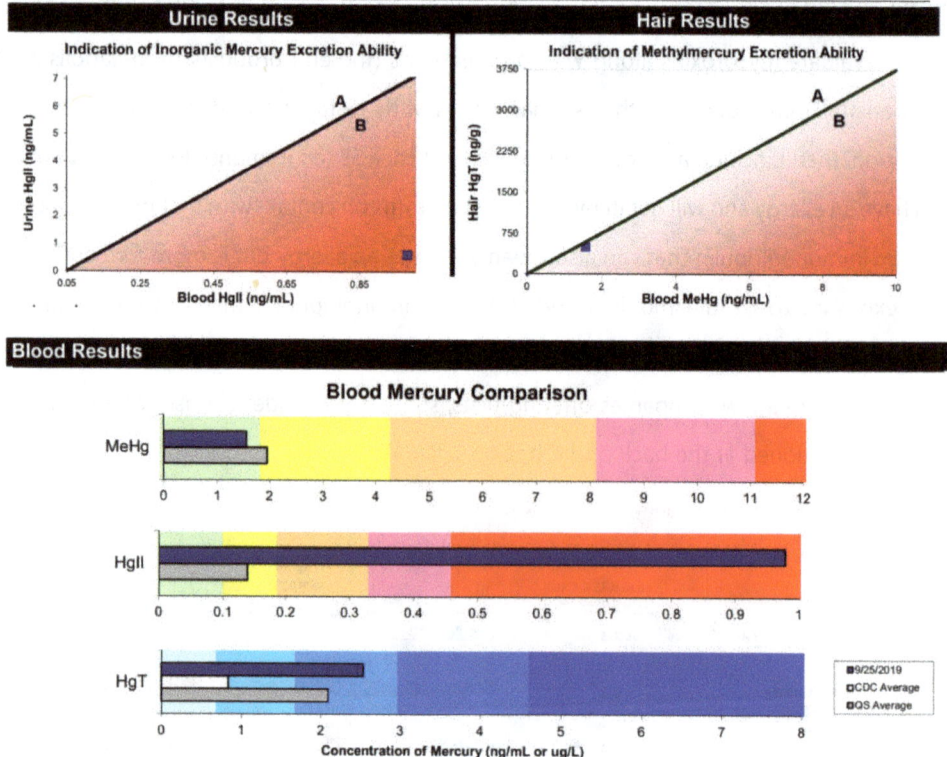

In the case above, we assessed hair, blood and urine in a single test. This patient had very high levels of mercury originating from dental fillings (HgII) and was also not detoxing well as seen by the back dot in the urine results (the red triangles), this should be on the black line if he was detoxing well. He had many alarming symptoms at this stage!

Blood tests for heavy metals can be done by any lab and are very useful for diagnosing lead toxicity, but unfortunately unless exposure is relatively recent, it isn't as useful for assessing the burden caused by other metals. Metals are considered very toxic by the body, so it tries to remove as much as possible as soon as possible, and anything it can't get rid of, it will store to be dealt with later. And as I mentioned, unless you are doing a biopsy on the exact tissue that the metal is stored in, you won't ever know the precise burden, so all these tests are more to evaluate the potential burden rather than to diagnose toxicity.

For persistent organic pollutants like plastics, testing becomes a little more complex due to the vast number of pollutants to test for any specifically. However, specialised labs are available to perform such tests if you want to test for them. I would recommend that you do the toxin exposure questionnaire at the end of the book. If you have lived near a source of exposure or eaten foods that are high-risk, then you can assume some amount of exposure. The good news is that all these toxins move out of the body in a similar way, so by reducing exposure, ensuring a healthy gut, and supporting the body through food, nutrition, sleep, exercise, sauna etc, you will still manage to get some, if not all, out eventually.

Essentially, if you suspect an environmental toxin is preventing you from healing, then test. Check your guts and then test for mycotoxins and moulds first, metals second, and finally POP's if you need to. Once you know the specific thing that is causing the problems, find the relevant reference chapter in this book and find out how you can remove it to make yourself a healthier version of yourself.

You can also test your response to stress (also a bad thing) and whether your stress glands, called the adrenals, need some love and support. My preference is to look at the active hormone in a 4-point saliva test along with a urinary assessment of the metabolites. This will give me a more complete picture of how much cortisol (the stress hormone we measure) is active versus how much is being made and used in total.

Keep following up with the questionnaires on the website and in the journal, to monitor your progress, and remember that it takes lots of good stuff, patience, and time to heal.

Chapter 4: What is the Good Stuff

The "Good Stuff" is anything that can assist with getting the bad stuff out, such as nutrients that can displace the bad stuff from the sites they are attached to, or life habits that can generally improve your health outcomes, such as good sleep, clean air, clean water and clean, nutritious food, less stress, more exercise and healthy relationships. As you now know, the human body was designed with its own systems to remove the bad stuff we are exposed to. Your liver, kidneys, skin, lungs, urinary and gut systems all work together to remove the unwanted harmful stuff that we encounter. That said, these systems still need some assistance from you due to the volume of stuff they have to deal with.

Nutrition	Exercise
Mitochondria	Stress management
Microbiome	Sauna therapy
Sleep	Self love

Nutrition and its role in detoxification

This topic is huge and has a few chapters dedicated to it, but essentially, your food choices and the nutrients you take can have a massive influence on your detoxification systems. The nutrients not only help your body to function and can displace stored bad stuff, but the foods you choose can also affect whether you absorb the bad stuff in the first place. Your food choices can also reduce the impact of the exposure to the bad stuff. Always choose your food well, then chew it very well!

Lets' start with the absorption of bad and good things from the gut. Absorption of bad metals is very much affected by your mineral content. In addition to mineral sufficiency, binding agents, or chelators, can be used to prevent absorption. Chelation is the bonding of organic molecules and metals that occurs naturally in the body, supported by enzymes such as metallothionein (MT) and a cofactor, such as essential vitamins and minerals. Examples of natural food chelators include chlorella and fucus and have been found to decrease mercury and lead in patients undergoing dental treatments.

Dietary sources of sulphur-containing foods (such as garlic and broccoli) are potential chelators as well. This is due to the toxic metal affinity for the nutrients in them. Sulphur-containing foods also increase glutathione production, which is a potent remover of bad things in general. Cilantro/coriander is another possible food chelator and has been shown to decrease heavy metal concentrations. There are some recipes on my website that include this ingredient, however, not everyone will enjoy the taste. There is a gene that makes some people taste this herb more as a soap than as something delicious!

Probiotics are becoming more widespread for their beneficial effect on the gut microbiota, and they are a potential tool to prevent damage in the gut caused by toxic metals. They have been shown to decrease toxic metal absorption in the gut due to improved binding, detoxification, and structural integrity. Sacchyromyces proboulardi is specifically good at binding to certain mycotoxins. If you are excited to learn more about the specifics, you can head over to the chapter titled 'A guide to using food as medicine'. Many nutrients are also covered in the chapters relating specifically to detoxification.

These are just the tip of the iceberg on the good stuff that good nutrients are, there is a whole section later that dives even deeper into what you should eat and why!

But for now, if you understand that food can be as effective as medicine, let's have a look at some of the other good things that we can support so that we can heal.

Mitochondria and Microbes and their role in detoxification and inflammation:

Very important good things are the bugs that live in and on us. Not the gross ones that cause disease, the good ones that prevent disease and give us energy. I am specifically referring to our mitochondria and microbiome. If we get the bad stuff out and feed the good bugs with good stuff, often that's already a few strands of the spiderweb being tugged on that will have a ripple effect of healing the body.

Let's start with the Mitochondria. I like to call them the "Mighty-chondria" because they are also known as the power cells or batteries of our cells! They create a molecule called Adenosine triphosphate (ATP) that, in most cases, helps us with energy. In 1967, a researcher named Lynn Margulis published a proposal that suggested that mitochondria were, in fact, bacteria that we have evolved to live with; in fact, we need them for the synthesis of ATP (energy); but they also need us as a safe home to live in.

The published article has led to cascade of subsequent articles stating that Mitochondria emerged from bacterial ancestors and have a very symbiotic relationship with us and are now crucial for cellular processes such as energy production and homeostasis (keeping the body in perfect balance), regulating the stress responses, cell survival, hormone regulation and more.

The symbiotic "agreement" that we seem to have with them is that we will house them and feed them good nutrients and keep them safe, and in turn, they will provide us with energy. This is important because, when we don't hold up our end of the bargain and they get exposed to heavy metals, mould etc., they stop providing the ATP molecules to us as energy and start using it to chat to each other as a warning that there are bad things encroaching on their homes! This is called the "cell danger response" and is one of the main reasons toxic exposure leads to fatigue and pain from the lack of functional ATP!

The Cell Danger Response (CDR) is a protective mechanism that occurs within our cells when the mitochondria sense various stressors, such as infections, injuries, toxins, or even psychological stress. It is a coordinated reaction aimed at promoting cell survival and restoring homeostasis (a balanced internal environment) in the face of potential harm.

Here's a brief explanation of the Cell Danger Response processes:

Recognition of Danger:

When the mitochondria sense a threat or danger, such as an infection or injury from toxins, they activate specific sensors that help the cells they live in detect various stress signals. These signals can come from damaged tissues, invading microorganisms, or other sources such as the bad stuff covered in this book.

Response Activation:

Once the danger is recognised, the cell triggers a series of protective responses to defend itself and restore normal function. These responses involve complex signalling pathways and cellular processes that use up the ATP we would usually have for energy.

Energy Redistribution:

During the CDR, cells prioritise energy allocation. They shift resources away from energy-consuming activities like growth and reproduction and redirect them towards processes that promote survival, repair, and defence. This can also contribute to the fatigue and brain fog people experience when burdened by bad stuff.

Inflammation:

Inflammation is a vital part of the CDR. It involves the release of chemical signals that attract immune cells to the affected area. Inflammation helps to remove harmful agents, clear cellular debris, and initiate tissue repair.

Immune Activation:

The immune system is mobilised as part of the CDR. Immune cells, such as white blood cells, are activated to eliminate pathogens, promote tissue healing, and restore a healthy balance. Unfortunately, inflammation often comes with pain!

Reprogramming and Adaptation:

The cell may undergo reprogramming to adapt to the stressor and protect itself from further damage. This reprogramming can involve changes in gene expression, protein production, and cellular processes to enhance survival and resilience.

Resolution and Recovery:

After eliminating or neutralising the threat, the CDR gradually diminishes. The body initiates the healing and recovery process to restore normal cell function and overall well-being. This is when we get our energy back.

Thankfully, there a couple of things you can do to help the Mitochondria resolve the CDR.

1 - Remove the source of the bad stuff.

2 - Feed the mitochondria well with both food and supplements when needed. Co-enzyme Q10, quercetin, NAD+ and pro resolving fatty acids like Omega 3, can all help. There are also many specific formulations on the market designed to improve mitochondrial health.

3 - Red light therapy is thought to supply the mitochondria with more energy.

Then there are the other bugs that form our extensive microbiome. There is a very famous saying that the gut is the "second brain," and you will find most practitioners who work in functional and lifestyle medicine will start by looking at the gut microbiome to assess its overall health. The microbiome is another group of bacteria that we also have an agreement with to home in a safe environment. If we don't feed the good gut bugs, then the bad gut bugs tend to start taking over, and then bad things happen to overall health. Oh, and the microbiome isn't just in the gut; there are specific microbiomes on our skin, in the different parts of our gut starting in the mouth and ending, well, at the end, and in women, there is even a microbiome in the vagina keeping things healthy! I am going to focus on the gut for now.

Imagine the gut as a long, hollow tube that is like a long doughnut hole going through you. It is one of the internal systems that has direct contact with the outside world. Because of this contact with the outside world being inside us, the gut houses about 70% of the immune system. It also changes PH (acidity and alkalinity) throughout and has different enzymes and bugs all the way through that should all be optimal for proper digestion and absorption of the foods we eat, and elimination of the things we don't want to have in us.

Sadly, for many people, a few things have gone slightly wrong over time. And I don't just mean the overuse of anti-biotics! Let me start with our lifestyles and the choices we are making about the foods to eat based on things like time, stress, and availability, instead of nourishment! The world we live in today has many easy-access foods to fit our very fast-paced lives. So, we choose foods based on time rather than nutritional value to the body. Then, also due to lack of time, we chew as few times as possible to get the food swallowed, practically inhaling the food. Unfortunately, chewing is a vital step in the digestive process. This action triggers what is called the "Cephalic" (Brain gets involved here) stage of digestion. During this stage, the brain sends signals to the stomach that food is on the way. The stomach then makes sure the acidity and enzymes are all ready for the proper digestion of the food. If this stage is missed, and we chew less, thanks to stress and time constraints, then the stomach isn't as prepared for the food as it should be, and the knock-on effect continues all the way through the rest of the tube, affecting the gut microbiome and us!

This makes another "Good thing", being mindful while eating and taking the time to chew your food well. Choose your food well and then, chew it well. Choose food that is the least processed, most nourishing and tasty as well as being food that will nourish not just you but also your mitochondria and your microbiome, then chew, chew and chew some more!

Practice this saying:

Drink your solids and chew your liquids.

This basically means chew your solids long enough so that they are liquid when you swallow them, and if you are drinking a smoothie, still have the action of chewing to improve the digestion and absorption of the good nutrients you have chosen! One task I give to people who really struggle with this, is to get a 30 second hourglass. They then must chew for as long as the sand is falling. They can have another bite when they turn the timer around again.

Healthy guts and gut bugs start in the mouth!

As mentioned before, I like to describe the guts as a long doughnut hole in the shape of a tube that goes from your mouth to your anus. This means that you need to be healthy from the mouth all the way through to the other end. Maintaining good oral health is paramount to the overall health of rest of the tube. It is important to always assess your mouth before embarking on a gut-healing program. Take a torch and have a good look in there! Is everything pink and healthy looking? Do your teeth look white and happy, are there any fillings, root canals, metals or infection? Remember that you may need to fix your mouth before moving on to removing any other bad things!

Let's talk toothpaste. As you may be aware, all ordinary toothpastes contain fluoride. While tiny doses that you don't swallow aren't going to cause any major disruption, the sad fact is that most people swallow a tube or more over their lifetime. There are alternatives readily available that contain botanicals and herbs that can clean the teeth. The occasional use of a charcoal-based toothpaste can also help, but be warned that it can also be abrasive, so don't use it every day. A better solution is a toothpaste that contains less fluoride and more nutrients like Co-enzyme Q10, calcium hydroxyapatite and probiotics. These are commercially available and can be used in conjunction with your normal toothpaste so that you reduce your exposure the fluoride.

It is also important to remember that you have a specific set of bacteria in your mouth that need to be kept happy! Heavy metals in the form of tooth fillings, caps, crowns etc., can upset the balance of these microbes, so please keep these metals to the bare minimum. Choose ceramic fillings, crowns, and avoid implants if possible. Make sure your gums are healthy, and that they don't bleed easily or get infected easily. Bleeding gums may mean you haven't got enough protein in your diet or that your oral microbiome is out of balance, get these assessed and back into balance so that the rest of your tube can stay happy. You can help those friendly mouth bugs by chewing a probiotic that is designed for oral health.

Probiotics are live bacteria and yeasts that have beneficial effects on your body. These species already live in your body, along with many others. Probiotic supplements add to your existing supply of friendly microbes. They help fight off the less friendly types and boost your immunity against infections. There is a lot of evidence to show that these good bugs can affect things like mental health as well as the gut, there is even evidence that when you don't have the good bugs you need, that you can increase your susceptibility to Parkinsons disease! Good gut bugs can be supplemented, but mostly, what they need is food! That comes from your food choices. They eat things called Pre-Biotics. You can eat chicory, dandelion greens, jerusalem artichoke, and other foods that have the right fibre content. Or you can take a prebiotic supplement.

Once you know your microbiome is happy and your guts are ready for active detoxification, go ahead and use what you need to get the bad stuff out, but don't forget that other lifestyle factors also need to be healthy, like sleep, exercise and the management of stress.

Sleep's role in detoxification and inflammation:

Sleep is totally under rated. In fact, I come from the generation of "I will sleep when I'm dead". Not me, I love to sleep! The term "beauty sleep" appeals to me more. Not only do you have a major antioxidant called Melatonin (the sleep hormone) upregulated during sleep, but Sleep also turns up the brains waste disposal system called the "Glymphatic System". During sleep, this system becomes more active and clears away toxins and waste products from the brain. At the same time, certain hormones are released that can help slow breathing and relax muscles. These sleep-inducing hormones can reduce inflammation in the body and support the detoxification process. As I mentioned, one essential hormone is Melatonin. This hormone is most related to the sleep side of our wake/sleep cycle, but it is way more than just a sleep hormone. It is also a very potent antioxidant and can help us to repair while we sleep! Antioxidants are very important, especially when you have been exposed to environmental toxins, which create oxidative stress and inflammation.

There is also a general increase in the activity of the liver and kidneys to improve detoxification while you sleep. When you sleep, your body isn't distracted by life and has a break from eating and drinking. That break means the liver and kidneys are enhanced to extract the bad stuff out of you. This is why I generally advise taking detox supplements and binders last thing at night. That way, whatever the liver processes in your sleep, gets supported and bound while you sleep!

Your quality of sleep can impact the levels of chemical messengers called cytokines, it can impact inflammatory markers, and even hormones. Lack of sleep can increase the levels of pro-inflammatory cytokines, which can contribute to chronic inflammation. Not sleeping well can also turn on 100's of pro inflammatory genes. These only get turned off once you have a few nights of good, restorative sleep. So essentially, sleep is anti-inflammatory.

Sleep is also crucial for supporting the immune system, which also plays an important role in inflammation. Adequate sleep can help regulate immune responses and promote the production of antibodies. Adequate sleep is necessary for overall health and well-being, and it's recommended that adults aim for 7-9 hours of sleep per night. If you're having trouble sleeping or are concerned about your sleep quality, it's best to consult with a healthcare professional for proper evaluation and guidance.

There are some habits, nutrients and herbs that can help if you are struggling with sleep. Here are some healthy sleep habits that can help improve your sleep quality:

1 - Stick to a Sleep Schedule:

Try to go to bed and wake up around the same time every day, even on weekends.

This helps regulate your body's internal clock and promotes better sleep.

2 - Create a Bedtime Routine:

Establish a relaxing routine before bed to signal to your body that it's time to sleep. This can include activities such as reading, taking a warm bath with epsom salts and aromatherapy oils, or practicing relaxation techniques.

3 - Get Regular Exercise:

Engage in regular physical activity during the day but avoid intense exercise close to bedtime. Exercise can help promote better sleep, but it's best to allow a few hours for your body to wind down before sleep.

4 - Create a Restful Environment:

Make your bedroom a sleep-friendly environment by keeping it cool, dark, and quiet. Use comfortable bedding and consider using earplugs, eye shades, or white noise machines if needed.

5 - Limit Daytime Naps:

If you have trouble sleeping at night, limit daytime napping or keep it short and early in the day. Avoid napping too close to your bedtime, as it can interfere with your ability to fall asleep at night.

6 - Pay Attention to Your Diet:

Be mindful of what you eat and drink, especially close to bedtime. Avoid heavy meals, caffeine, nicotine, and alcohol, as they can disrupt sleep patterns.

7 - Manage Stress:

Practice stress management techniques, such as relaxation exercises, meditation, or journaling, to help calm your mind before bed.

8 - Create a Comfortable Sleep Environment:

Invest in a comfortable mattress, pillows, and bedding that support your sleep needs. Ensure that your bedroom is free from distractions and electronic devices.

Remember, everyone's sleep needs are different, so it's important to find what works best for you. If you continue to experience sleep difficulties, it's recommended to consult with a healthcare professional for further evaluation and guidance.

If you are still struggling, then you can try one of the following:

Calcium and *Magnesium:*

These are both minerals that play a role in muscle and nerve function Their significant role in promoting relaxation and reducing stress makes them potential contributors to better sleep quality.

Hops, Poppy, Valerian Root Passionflower and Holy Basil:

These herbs have been used for centuries as natural sleep aids. They may help improve sleep quality and reduce the time it takes to fall asleep.

L-Theanine:

This is an amino acid found in tea leaves that may help promote relaxation and reduce stress. It may help improve sleep quality by promoting relaxation and reducing anxiety.

5-HTP:

Some studies suggest that 5-HTP may improve sleep quality and reduce the time it takes to fall asleep. It is believed to increase the production of serotonin, which can be converted into melatonin, a hormone that regulates sleep.

Glycine:

Glycine is another amino acid that has been shown to help sleep. Taking glycine helps you reach deep sleep more quickly and improves your quality of sleep by stabilising your sleep rhythms and as a bonus, it tastes sweet too.

If you are still struggling, then please see a functional medicine practitioner.

Exercise's role in detoxification and inflammation:

Exercise promotes blood circulation, which can help the liver and lymph do their job of removing toxins from the body. Your lymphatic system is a group of organs, vessels and tissues that protect you from infection and keep a healthy balance of fluids throughout your body. It is another way the body removes the bad stuff. Lymphatic system organs include your bone marrow, thymus and lymph nodes. Unlike the cardiovascular system that has a heart pumping the blood around, your lymphatic system doesn't have a heart to pump the lymph fluid around, it relies on muscles contracting to move the lymph. Exercise also increases sweat production, which can help release more bad stuff from the body. Sweating plays an especially important role in the removal of environmental pollutants, mycotoxins and heavy metals.

Exercise has also been shown to help control inflammation in the body. Although inflammation is a natural and necessary immune response, chronic inflammation is harmful to the body and can contribute to various health problems. Exercise can help reduce inflammation and support overall health. The type and intensity of exercise can impact its effects on detoxification and inflammation. Low-intensity aerobic exercise that increases the heart rate and causes heavier breathing is a recommended detox method, as is something simple like gently jumping on a trampoline, called rebounding. My advice is to find a sport you enjoy and get your exercise doing that. That way you experience the joy in movement which would also improve your responses to stress.

Infra-red sauna therapy:

The use of near, far, and mid infra-red rays helps to encourage sweating, one of the ways we remove the bad stuff. During an infrared sauna session, the heat generated by the sauna penetrates deep into the tissues, stimulating blood flow and metabolic activity. This process is known as hyperthermia, which promotes the release of toxins from the body via natural sweating and increased tissue oxygenation.

The sauna encourages cardiovascular health with new oxygenated blood flow to cells to help reduce inflammation caused by mould, mycotoxins, heavy metals and POP's. The heat waves penetrate the skin more deeply than traditional saunas, allowing for the removal of a more significant amount of toxins.

Infrared sauna therapy has been shown to increase levels of heat shock proteins, which help repair damaged cells and enhance immune function. Additionally, infrared heat therapy has been shown to decrease inflammation markers and support respiratory function, potentially improving some of the symptoms associated with toxicity.

To get the most out of your infrared sauna sessions, follow these tips:

Hydration:

Drink plenty of water before and after each sauna session to stay hydrated and facilitate toxin elimination. Feel free to add electrolytes.

Gradual Increase:

Start with shorter sauna sessions and gradually increase the duration to prevent overexposure and potential side effects. It is essential to note that any potential side effects usually are from mould exposure, not the infrared sauna therapy itself.

Lifestyle Changes:

Lifestyle changes such as adopting a healthy diet, regular exercise, and stress management can support your body's healing process and detoxification efficiency.

If you're new to infrared saunas or have any medical conditions, it's always best to consult a healthcare provider beforehand. Once in the sauna, start with lower temperatures and shorter session times, gradually working your way up as your body becomes more acclimated to the heat. Remember to listen to your body and exit the sauna if you feel lightheaded or uncomfortable at any point. And if you can't sauna, break a sweat through exercise!

Managing stress can improve detoxification processes in the body:

When experiencing stress, people often resort to self-medication, such as consuming alcohol or sweet sugary foods. In this way, stress can contribute to the accumulation of bad things in the body. By managing stress, people can reduce their toxic load and support the body's natural detoxification processes. Chronic stress can also contribute to inflammation in the body, interfering with detoxification processes. By managing stress, you can reduce inflammation and support overall health.

Some ways to manage stress and support detoxification processes include:

- Regular exercise, such as yoga/tai chi, aerobic exercise, rebounding or stretching
- Mindfulness practices, such as meditation
- Adequate sleep and rest
- Journalling.
- Therapy
- Breathing! So many people have forgotten how to breathe properly!

Breathing reduces stress, so try this exercise:

This calming breathing technique for stress, anxiety and panic takes just a few minutes and can be done anywhere. You will get the most benefit if you do it regularly, as part of your daily routine.

You can do it standing up, sitting in a chair that supports your back, or lying on a bed or mat on the floor. Make yourself as comfortable as you can. If you can, loosen any clothes that restrict your breathing.

If you're lying down, place your arms a little bit away from your sides, with the palms up. Let your legs be straight or bend your knees so your feet are flat on the floor. If you're sitting, place your arms on the chair arms.

If you're sitting or standing, place both feet flat on the ground. Whatever position you're in, place your feet roughly hip-width apart.

Let your breath flow as deep down into your belly as is comfortable, without forcing it.

Breathe in through your nose and out through your mouth.

Breathe in gently and regularly. Some people find it helpful to count steadily from 1 to 5. You may not be able to reach 5 at first.

Then let it flow out gently, counting from 1 to 5 again.

Keep doing this for at least 5 minutes.

Self-Love

This is covered in the chapter on toxic people, but essentially, you need to kind and patient with yourself as you heal. No one does things perfectly. It takes practice to learn new habits. There is no one way to do things correctly, so trust yourself. Remember, that if you can't love and respect yourself and your ability to heal, this will affect your healing.

Summary:

- Make good choices for your microbes and mitochondria
- Eat, drink, and breathe clean
- Maintain good oral and overall gut health
- Be mindful while eating (tip - don't be watching TV or on your phone)
- Chew your feed VERY well
- Sleep well
- Get some form of movement daily
- Practice stress management
- Breathe
- Sauna
- Remember to be kind to yourself as you heal

Chapter 5: What Does It Feel Like to Heal

If you or someone you know, or someone you are treating is about to embark on their healing journey, then consider this critical discussion that I recommend you have with them, about the healing process.

Healing, especially from chronic conditions caused by exposure to bad things in our environment, is not a linear journey of being sick one day, being on a program and at the end of the program, suddenly feeling better. The general expectation is that once you start putting the good stuff in, such as good nutrients, good movement, improved sleep, stress management and even improved relationships; that you will experience an amazing and immediate transformation to being 100% healthy. Sadly, this is not the case. Also, more irritatingly, what you (or the person being treated) think should be resolved first may be the last thing to improve. The reason for this is that the body will triage nutrients to the areas it knows need to be fixed first, meaning that your body will send the good stuff where it KNOWS is a priority, not where you THINK is a priority. I can't tell you how often the people with acne, hair loss, or weight gain, only see the results they want, after many other organ systems have started to improve. This is why I highly recommend tracking and journaling.

I always explain to my patients that the healing journey will have ups and downs starting from day 1. In fact, I warn them that they may feel periods of feeling worse for a few days and then feel better and then worse again. If they have many layers of bad stuff, their body, in its immense intelligence, will decide which toxin to remove first, regardless of which one you may think is most important!

My best advice is to start slowly on any program, build up to doses that are easily tolerated, that will be effective, and most importantly, TRUST & BE PATIENT with the process... it takes time to remove stored stuff, and they may have had years of exposure.

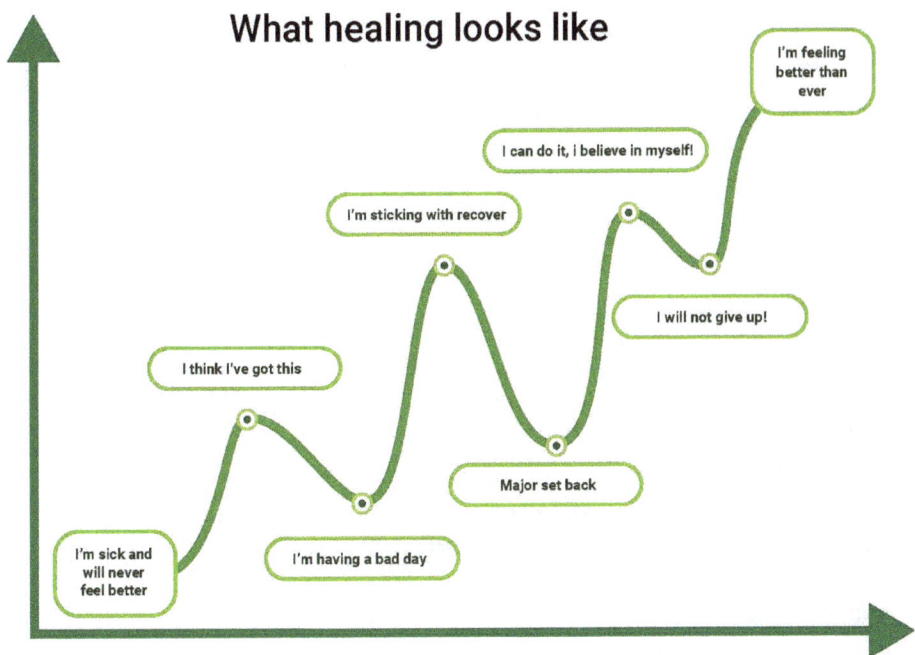

In my programs, I always treat the environment first. That means purifying the air and water and choosing good quality food and supplements. Once that is done, they can start on themselves.

Here are some stories/tips that I tell people to help them cope with the uncomfortableness that comes with healing:

Goldfish analogy for exposure:

You can't heal in the same environment that made you sick, and you wouldn't expect a goldfish to be healthy in a dirty fishbowl. Clean your environment first.

Trust your body's ability to heal:

If you break a bone, it won't be broken forever, but it also doesn't heal overnight, it takes time. In the case of a long-term chronic exposure that resulted in chronic disease, it will take even more time. And it is uncomfortable, itchy, annoying and often frustrating. When they express their frustration, which they always do, I remind them with the diagram, just where they are on their journey.

I give them a task:

They need to plant a seed and nurture it to the point it bears fruit; that is roughly the time they need to give themselves to heal before they can complain about the time it takes to heal. Be patient with the process.

The good news is that, throughout the journey, there will always be improvements even within the dips and flares. It isn't the case that you feel awful and then spontaneously feel better a year into the process, there will be gradual improvements along the way.

Common symptoms experienced:

Common symptoms experienced:
1. A return of old symptoms, but then they leave as per the tip below
2. Changes in bowel habits; these are also transitory
3. In women, changes in the menstrual cycle
4. Random joint pains and muscle aches
5. Flu or hangover-like symptoms
6. Headaches and brain fog that comes and goes
7. Flares ups in skin conditions, increased dryness, acne etc.
8. Moodiness and a desire to cry for no reason

The 4 day "flare"

Few people are aware of this, but as your body mobilises anything, like a heavy metal or a mycotoxin from wherever it is stored in the body, it moves out that stored tissue and into the bloodstream. When this happens, there is a 4 day "flare up" of their symptoms.

Let's look at a scenario where someone was exposed to more bad stuff than their body could cope with. In this case, the body would put the surplus stuff that the liver couldn't cope with, into storage. Usually into fatty tissue, but sometimes into bones and other organs.

Now they have rehabilitated their environment and removed the source of exposure. They have also changed some habits and now their body is able to spring clean that stuff out of them. To do this, that stored stuff is taken out of storage and is slowly processed by the detox organ systems. This mobilisation of most toxins generally results in a **4 day "flare up"** or aggravation of symptoms; the exception of this would be mycotoxins, where the flares can last as long as 10 days. The symptoms in these 4-10 days vary depending on which toxin is being mobilised and that is prioritised by the body.

My tip to my patients, is to celebrate these 4 days and when they are experienced, because they have removed another layer of bad stuff and to remind them that this is what actual healing feels like!

An example of what a flare might feel like is, if the heavy metal lead (Pb) is being mobilised, the joints will hurt lot, but won't be hot, just sore. Gut motility may slow down, making they feel possibly constipated and generally unwell.

If the heavy metal mercury (Hg) is being mobilised, then brain fog worsens, and dizziness and other neurological symptoms flare up.

But only for 4 days.

Another point to remember, is that the body deals with stored stuff in waves, so there will be 4 days of flare ups, followed by ANY amount of time; days, week, even months might pass until the next wave is dealt with. This all depends on the program they are on, what steps have been put in place and a variety of other factors.

Herings law of cure

Founded by Constantine Hering, M.D. Hering's Law of Cure is considered important to the philosophy of complementary medicines such as naturopathy. It suggests that healing occurs with a distinct and consistent pattern.

Positive healing symptoms according to Hering's law include aggravations or 'healing crisis', new 'healing symptoms and the systematic return of old symptoms.

Based on the principle of Hering's Law these symptoms should reflect the following patterns of cure:

From the Head Down:

Symptoms improve from the head down, for example a skin rash may move towards the hands, or a sore throat may heal before a sore knee further down the body.

From the inside out:

During healing the disease or stored bad stuff, needs to leave the body from internal organs outwards. This may manifest in excessive sweat, loose bowel movements, excessive mucous production or frequent urination. This response can be quite rapid and is sometimes termed as a healing crisis. These tend to last about 4 days when you are mobilising heavy metals.

From the most important organs to the least important:

The body will first express the deepest symptoms in the most important organs (the lungs or liver) because they are the greatest threat to the life force. This healing response may subsequently result in the symptoms moving to an organ of lesser importance such as the skin.

In the reverse order of symptoms that they first appeared:

During healing, previous diseases that have been suppressed when a worse disease comes along, may reappear; this can be seen as a healing crisis. For example, a patient who suffered childhood eczema, later developed hay fever then finally asthma, may see their hay fever return followed by eczema as healing progresses.

Explain the process to anyone wanting to embark on a healing journey. Keep these principles in mind, especially on the days where the symptoms feel worse, not better... those days will pass, and you will recover. You just need the good stuff to outweigh the bad and of course, time. Healing is possible with the right ingredients, the right mindset and time!

Chapter 6: Prepping for Detoxification and Covering the Bases

If you are anything like me, when I realised, I was toxic, all I wanted was for those toxins to be out... NOW! Unfortunately, this is not a healthy way to think about or support your process. Remember that you are like the spider in a web and too much stimulation is not good. There are steps that need to be taken to ensure you are healthy through the process and that you don't damage yourself even more. Once you have removed the source of the bad stuff, you can then prepare yourself for active removal of that bad stuff.

Always make sure you CAN detox. We detox via pooping, peeing, and sweating predominantly. Please make sure you are not constipated before starting any kind of detox. If you are, then that needs to be fixed first! If you don't sweat well, then assess and support that too. Your liver and kidneys will also be placed under some strain while mobilising metals and mycotoxins, so please ensure that they are up for the job. And, of course, don't forget; you need healthy guts for healthy detoxification.

Before you do anything with your body, make sure you reduce your burden by reducing exposure. Have your home assessed for mould but a qualified professional. Clean your air with a dehumidifier and air purifier, clean your water with a water purifier, and choose to eat clean, healthy, nutritious food. Start with improving your diet.

Let's chat about food again for a minute, so you can prep your kitchen:

Protein

Protein is an essential macronutrient, but not all food sources of protein are created equal. Protein is a nutrient your body needs to grow and repair cells, and to work properly.

Protein is found in a wide range of food and it's important that you get enough protein in your diet every day. How much protein you need from your diet varies depending on your weight, gender, age and health.

Prioritise protein at each meal. Protein breaks down into amino acids, and healthy detoxification needs these amino acids to bind to the bad stuff so you can remove them. Protein also helps your tissues to repair and heal. Proteins mostly come from animal sources, but vegetables contain some as well, so you can mix them up a bit. If you are vegan or vegetarian, please consider supplementing protein while actively removing bad stuff. Protein is primarily digested in the mouth and stomach. Always remember to chew, chew and chew, so that when the protein enters the stomach it is closer to being amino acids (the smallest thing it can be) and absorption is better.

Meeting your protein needs is easily achieved from eating a variety of foods:

Regeneratively farmed free range meats:

Free range poultry like duck, chicken or turkey and cuts of free-range beef, lamb, and pork are excellent sources of protein. Choose grass fed meat as it contains a better balance of omega 3 than grain fed meat. If you have chosen to be vegetarian or vegan, please obviously use vegetable sources listed instead.

Fish and Seafood:

Fish and seafood are rich in protein and often provide additional health benefits due to their omega-3 fatty acid content. Examples include salmon, tuna, trout, sardines, shrimp, and cod. If you are worried about heavy metals, reduce your consumption of "fish that eat other fish" like tuna, barracuda and swordfish, but also reduce shellfish as they may also have high metals as unfortunately shellfish and predatory fish can contain a higher number of heavy metals in their bodies. Wild-caught salmon, trout, krill, shrimp, crayfish, lobster, crab, red seabream, crawfish, and salmon roe contains a wonderful substance called Astaxanthin. A bioflavonoid that can help protect against damage from oxidative stress. Please note that farm-raised fish get their astaxanthin resources through commercially made food additives containing synthetic astaxanthin, which is made from petrochemicals, so they are NOT the same thing!

Eggs:

Eggs are a nutrient-dense source of protein, providing all the essential amino acids our body needs. They also contain nutrients like choline and beta carotene that would support the body. They are also versatile and can be prepared in various ways, such as boiled, scrambled, or poached. Avoid if you have any intolerance to eggs.

Dairy Products:

Dairy products such as milk, yogurt, and cheese are good sources of protein, particularly casein and whey proteins. Reduce or avoid dairy if you have any sensitivity to it or have lactose intolerance. Follow the advice of your healthcare provider when it comes to dairy intolerance.

Legumes:

Legumes, including beans, lentils, and peas, are excellent plant-based sources of protein. They are also high in fibre, making them a nutritious choice.

Tofu and Tempeh:

Tofu and tempeh are soy-based products and popular protein sources for vegetarians and vegans. They are versatile ingredients that can be used in various recipes and dishes.

Nuts and Seeds:

While not as high in protein as animal-based sources, nuts and seeds provide a good amount of protein along with healthy fats and other nutrients. However, if you are specifically detoxing mould, you may want to avoid these until you are better, as they tend to attract mould.

Quinoa and Other Whole Grains:

Quinoa is a unique plant-based protein source that also contains all the essential amino acids, and this is why it is included throughout the Reset program. Other whole grains like brown rice, oats, and whole wheat products also contribute to protein intake. Many people who are burdened with toxins are also grain intolerant, especially wheat, so if you are inflamed and toxic, you may want to reduce these until you feel better.

Whey and Plant-Based Protein Powders:

Protein powders, such as whey, pea protein, hemp protein, or rice protein, can be convenient options for boosting protein intake, particularly for individuals following vegetarian or vegan diets.

Carbohydrates in the form of Food & Vegetables

Next you should prioritise your plant-based nutrients. I recommend making sure you get enough of a plant group that contains a substance called bioflavonoids. These are a group of plant compounds that are believed to have a range of health benefits, including antioxidant and anti-inflammatory effects. Some flavonoids, such as apigenin and luteolin, can reduce the mycotoxin citrinin. Bioflavonoids can also reduce the build-up of toxins from the mould Aspergillus flavus. They also have antioxidant effects, which can help protect against free radical damage caused by mycotoxins and other toxins.

Bioflavonoids are found in many fruits and vegetables, including citrus fruits, berries, apples, grapes, pomegranates, plums, and red wine. They are also found in vegetables such as celery, parsley, herbs, peppers, onions, leeks, brussels sprouts, kale, and broccoli. Bioflavonoids are active ingredients in many herbal remedies, including feverfew, ginkgo biloba, and liquorice root. I suggest to my patients that they eat 5-7 servings of vegetables every day and try to eat a different vegetable from the full colour palette each meal– green, orange, purple, yellow, red, blue – the whole rainbow. In fact, aim to eat 20 different vegetables every week to make sure you get the variety you need. It's best to keep your fruit intake to a minimum at the beginning of treatment to prevent fungal overgrowth (but if you're having a sweet craving, fruit is better than all-out sugar.) Remember that herbal teas are better than coffee when detoxing and can help add more bioflavonoids!

Please moderate the red wine and the very sweet fruit! Too much sugar can make a mould colony very happy and negate the positive effects of bioflavonoids! You can also get bioflavonoids in the form of supplements. Look for astaxanthin, pycnogenol, lutein, Polyphenol-C, quercetin, and grape seed extract, to name a few.

Here is a list of some foods that are rich in bioflavonoids:
Berries, including strawberries, raspberries, blueberries, and blackberries
Citrus fruits, including oranges, lemons, and limes
Apples, grapes, pomegranates, plums
Red wine, but limited if you are detoxing
Vegetables, including celery, parsley, herbs, peppers, onions, leeks, brussels sprouts, kale and broccoli, but try to eat all the colours daily!
Soybeans and legumes

Cocoa and green tea
Many spices, including turmeric

Fats

Many toxins are what are called Lipophilic, which means, they get stored in fat. To ensure that they get removed, you basically need to service your oil and change it up, like you would for your car, to maintain its health. To do this you need to make sure you are eating healthy fats at every meal. The most researched and one of my favourites, it is good quality, extra virgin olive oil and you can eat this as much as you want to. How do you know it's good quality? Well, if you taste a little, your tongue should tingle slightly; that's a sign of the active plant ingredients called polyphenols, working! The other good oils tend to come in solid food form, like avocados, flax/linseeds, sunflower, and pumpkin seeds, or wild-caught oily fish or grass-fed red meat (yes, grass-fed red meat contains omega 3, a very healthy fat). Avoid too many sources of refined seed oils and grain-fed meats, they are much higher in Omega 6, which isn't always bad, but it is not good when you want to balance the intake of Omega 3!

Bile flow stimulators (Cholagogues)

At this stage of preparation, you can also start eating more foods that support bile flow and overall detoxification. Toxins go through the liver and get packaged in bile, so ensuring a happy, healthy flow of bile is essential. Bile is a vital body fluid that plays an important role in the absorption of nutrients in the small intestine as well as in flushing the liver of toxins. Bile is continuously produced in the liver by cholesterol bound to 2 amino acids called glycine and taurine. It is then stored in the gallbladder. Bile salts break down fats, so adequate bile is required for processing fats. Bile also transports toxins out of the liver into the poop and keeps everything flowing.

Here are some foods and drinks that can help support healthy bile flow;

All dark green leafy vegetables, beetroot, artichokes, pickles, roasted dandelion root tea, lemon tea, celery juice, and coffee are great at stimulating bile production.

Celery, radish, artichokes, high-fat diet, foods with certain types of fat like polyunsaturated fat, avocados, fatty fish like salmon, nuts like cashews and almonds, garlic, onions, grapefruits, and vegetable juicing with bitter green veggies.

Eat a high-fibre and high-protein diet with lots of vegetables, legumes, and nuts. Drink plenty of water as bile is primarily composed of it. If you're dehydrated, your bile production will suffer.

Try food before supplements, but if you still feel you need support, then supplements like Swedish bitters, choline, glycine, and taurine in a supplement form can help build bile.

Herbs, such as Triphala, shilajit, guduchi, hibiscus, fenugreek seeds, cinnamon stick, turmeric, and ginger, can also help.

Binders

Next, you can start adding foods that act as binders. These will bind to bile and the toxins in the gut, so you can poop then out rather than reabsorb them. Psyllium fibre and glucomannan can bind to bile acids and toxins in the intestines. Raisin dietary fibre has also been shown to be an effective binder. However, be aware that dried fruits are best avoided when you have mould or mycotoxins. Overall, consuming fibre-rich foods can have a positive impact on bile acid binding and removal from the body. Examples of supplemental binders include N-Acetyl cysteine, sacchyromyces boulardi (a probiotic), activated charcoal, various clays, silica, apple pectin, and aloe. Pharmaceutical binders are also available, you can discuss these with your practitioner as they will need to be prescribed.

Nucleotides

Then there is the often-missed food group called Nucleotides. Nucleotides are micronutrients that serve as the building blocks of DNA and RNA, which contain our genetic information. They are essential for various biological processes in the body, including cell division and the production of proteins, enzymes, neurotransmitters, hormones, and other body chemicals. The problem is we get very little from our diet these days as so few people enjoy organ meats, which contain the highest available amount. Vegetarians and vegans get even less through diet as very few plant sources of nucleotides exist. Luckily, they can be supplemented, so keep an eye out for them if you don't get enough from food!

Eating or supplementing nucleotides can have potential health benefits, including:

Advanced Recovery:

Nucleotide-supplemented diets have been shown to improve the composition of the liver and aid in recovery, even after severe mycotoxin exposure.

Gut Repair:

Nucleotides can support gut health by reducing cortisol levels and increasing secretory IgA, which is important for immune function

Immune Support:

Nucleotides can strengthen the acquired immune system, helping to resist the invasion of pathogenic bacteria and reducing the risk of infections.

Protein Synthesis:

Nucleotides are essential for protein synthesis, making them beneficial for increasing muscle tone and supporting muscle recovery.

Stress Reduction:

Dietary nucleotides have been found to reduce the release of stress-related hormones and chemicals in the body, potentially helping to mitigate the negative health impacts of stress.

The best food sources of nucleotides include:

Meat: Meat, such as beef, pork, and chicken, is considered one of the richest sources of nucleotides, containing 1.5-8 grams of nucleic acids per 3.5 ounces (100 grams)

Fish: Fish is another excellent source of nucleotides, providing 1.5-8 grams of nucleic acids per 3.5 ounces (100 grams). It is also a good source of protein, omega-3 fats, vitamin D, selenium, and iodine.

Organ Meats: Organ meats, like liver and heart, are particularly high in nucleotides. They are considered among the most abundant sources of nucleotides in adult diets.

Seafood: Seafood, including shellfish, is a good source of nucleotides. While it provides slightly smaller amounts compared to meat and fish, it remains a nutritious option.

Vegetables including: celery, parsley, herbs, peppers, onions, leeks, brussels sprouts, kale and broccoli, but try to eat all the colours daily!

Beans, Lentils, and Peas: Legumes, such as beans, lentils, and peas, are plant-based sources of nucleotides. They can be beneficial for vegans and vegetarians, but the amount of nucleotides is still very low in comparison to animal sources, and I would recommend additional supplementation.

Milk and Dairy Products: Milk and dairy products may contain significant amounts of nucleotides. However, the concentration may vary depending on processing.

After addressing your kitchen, the next step in preparation would be to make sure your oral health is good.

Stand in front of a mirror and have a look at your gums and tongue. Note any changes in colour, infections, receding gums, root canals, crowns, and fillings. If you have metal fillings (the old silver ones in particular), consider removing them before you start anything. Removal needs to be done by a dentist who understands heavy metals. A dental dam MUST be used, and the filling should ideally be replaced with a natural composite rather than white metals. Patients who are concerned about the potential health risks associated with dental fillings should speak with their dentist about natural and non-toxic options.

If you noted any changes in colour, tongue coating, infections etc., please seek health from a qualified provider to assist you. There is a guide in the journal that can help you with this.

Finally, before proceeding, you could do some preliminary blood work that would include:

- Liver function test
- Kidney function tests including uric acid
- Full blood count to assess the red and white blood cells
- Thyroid function test

If you can, then also do a microbiome analysis of your poop.

Once you have all these bases covered, improved your diet, made sure you can detox in a healthy way, then you can move on to actively mobilising the bad stuff.

Chapter 7: Important Vitamins and Co-Factors

In the chapter where I go into why heavy metals are specifically bad, I will mention that when thinking of heavy metals and nutritional metals, I like to think of them as a large family, the relationships will be discussed more in their reference section but essentially they are the close family members where some get along, some don't and it is their relationships that affect us.

When it comes to vitamins and co-factors, they are also a part of that family, like cousins and more distant relatives. As they are still part of the family, some members of the vitamin family help the other mineral family members work a bit better, and sometimes, if they aren't there, nothing gets done!

Nutrient co-factors are substances that work together with other nutrients to enhance their absorption, bioavailability, or effectiveness in the body. They play important roles in various biochemical processes and are necessary for optimal health. Here are some common nutrient co-factors:

Vitamin D and Calcium:

Vitamin D facilitates the absorption of calcium and phosphorus in the intestines and supports its utilisation in the body. These two nutrients work together to maintain strong bones and teeth.

Vitamin C and Iron:

Vitamin C enhances the absorption of non-haem iron, the type of iron found in plant-based foods. Eating vitamin C-rich foods alongside iron-rich foods can help improve iron absorption.

Vitamin B12 and Folate:

Vitamin B12 and folate are both involved in red blood cell production and DNA synthesis. They have interdependent roles, and deficiencies in one can affect the function of the other. It's important to maintain adequate levels of both nutrients for optimal health.

Vitamin E and Selenium:

Vitamin E and selenium are antioxidants that work together to protect cells from oxidative damage. Selenium helps to regenerate vitamin E, enhancing its antioxidant activity in the body.

Zinc and Vitamin A:

Zinc is necessary for the metabolism and utilisation of vitamin A. Adequate zinc levels are required for the conversion of the precursor form of vitamin A (beta-carotene) into its active form.

Magnesium and Vitamin D:

Magnesium is involved in the activation and metabolism of vitamin D. Adequate magnesium levels are important for optimal vitamin D function and utilisation in the body.

Vitamin K and Vitamin D:

Vitamin K plays a crucial role in the activation of certain proteins involved in blood clotting and bone metabolism. Vitamin D helps regulate calcium levels, and vitamin K is required for the proper utilisation of calcium in the body, ensuring that the vitamin D is deposited into bones and not soft tissue.

Choline:

Choline is a nutrient that is found in many foods. Your brain and nervous system need it to regulate memory, mood, muscle control, and other functions. You also need choline to form the membranes that surround your body's cells. Choline plays a very important role in detoxing mycotoxins.

Coenzyme Q10 (CoQ10):

CoQ10 acts with many nutrients and is considered a potent co-factor in nutrition. CoQ10 is a naturally occurring compound found in almost all cells in the body and plays a crucial role in energy production within the mitochondria, often referred to as the "powerhouse" of cells. CoQ10 acts as a co-factor or coenzyme for several enzymes involved in the cellular energy production process. CoQ10 is not only involved in energy metabolism but also functions as a potent antioxidant, protecting cells from oxidative damage. It works in conjunction with other antioxidants, such as vitamin E, to neutralise harmful free radicals.

Co-factors play a vital role in the manufacture of energy. The Krebs cycle, also known as the citric acid cycle or the tricarboxylic acid (TCA) cycle, is a series of chemical reactions that occur in the mitochondria of cells. It is an essential part of cellular respiration and energy production. Several co-factors play important roles in the Krebs cycle, facilitating the enzymatic reactions and allowing for the efficient conversion of nutrients into energy.

Here are some of the key co-factors involved in the Krebs cycle:

Vitamin B3 - **NAD+ (Nicotinamide adenine dinucleotide)**:

NAD stands for Nicotinamide. Adenine Dinucleotide is a form of Vitamin B3. NAD+ is a co-factor that carries electrons during various reactions in the Krebs cycle. It accepts electrons from the oxidation of molecules, such as isocitrate and alpha-ketoglutarate, and is reduced to NADH. NADH then participates in the electron transport chain, ultimately leading to the production of ATP (adenosine triphosphate).

Vitamin B2 - **FAD (Flavin adenine dinucleotide):**

FAD is a coenzyme form of vitamin B2 and another co-factor that carries electrons during specific reactions in the Krebs cycle. It accepts electrons from the oxidation of succinate, forming FADH2. Like NADH, FADH2 participates in the electron transport chain to generate ATP (energy).

Vitamin B5 - **Coenzyme A (CoA)**:

Pantothenate is vitamin B5 and is the key precursor for the biosynthesis of coenzyme A (CoA), a universal and essential cofactor involved in a myriad of metabolic reactions, including the synthesis of phospholipids, the synthesis and degradation of fatty acids, and the operation of the tricarboxylic acid cycle. Coenzyme A plays a crucial role in the Krebs cycle by forming acetyl-CoA, a molecule that enters the cycle. Acetyl-CoA is derived from the breakdown of glucose, fatty acids, and amino acids, and it combines with oxaloacetate to initiate the cycle.

Vitamin B1 - **Thiamine pyrophosphate (TPP):**

TPP is derived from vitamin B1 (thiamine) and serves as a co-factor for the enzyme pyruvate dehydrogenase, which catalyses the conversion of pyruvate to acetyl-CoA. Acetyl-CoA is then used as a substrate in the Krebs cycle.

Lipoic acid:

Lipoic acid acts as a co-factor for the enzyme complex called pyruvate dehydrogenase complex, which helps convert pyruvate into acetyl-CoA. It also participates in the oxidation of alpha-ketoglutarate in the Krebs cycle.

These co-factors, along with other enzymes and substrates, work together in the Krebs cycle to generate energy-rich molecules like NADH and FADH2, which feed into the electron transport chain to produce ATP. The Krebs cycle is a complex and interconnected series of reactions, and the co-factors play vital roles in facilitating the efficient flow of energy production within cells.

Even though it can get complicated, I hope that you can see how vital these nutrients, minerals, vitamins, and co-factors are in keeping yourself healthy in this modern world. Without these vital ingredients, you won't be able to create energy, detoxify, and reduce inflammation and oxidative stress, meaning that you will develop symptoms without them. This is why you should always ensure a good intake of these nutrients through a healthy, balanced diet and, where needed, supplements. It's worth noting that nutrient interactions and co-factors can be complex, and the examples mentioned above are just a few of many possible interactions. A well-balanced and varied diet that includes a wide range of nutrient-rich foods can help ensure adequate intake of co-factors and support optimal nutrient absorption and utilisation. If you have specific concerns or questions about nutrient co-factors, it's best to consult with a healthcare professional, registered nutritional therapist, or dietitian.

Chapter 8: Diving Deeper into Detoxification & Dealing with The Bad Stuff

This chapter gets a little geeky, so you can skip it if you just want to know how to remove your identified bad stuff by using the reference sections later in the book.

Detoxification is far from simple, but it is a finely oiled machine that is excellent at its job. Our body's innate system of recycling and taking out the trash is PROFOUND. We need to be reminded to trust our body's ability to heal itself! Most of this occurs without any intervention, but with a world increasing in toxins by the second, our systems are becoming burdened, and some support is now often required.

For those of you who are not aware of the internal mechanisms we have in place to remove toxicants, this chapter should help shed some light on those processes.

We have specific systems in place to help reduce our toxic load. To simplify the phases of detoxification, I will refer to them as linear processes moving from 0-3. However, all these processes are happening all at once in the body.

Generally speaking, addressing Phase 0 (reducing or removing the exposure), ignoring Phase 1 and supporting Phase 2 and Phase 3 detoxification can be powerful tools, but even if you are a qualified practitioner treating yourself, before beginning any detox and supplement regimen, I strongly recommend working with a physician who can help you understand your body's specific needs objectively!

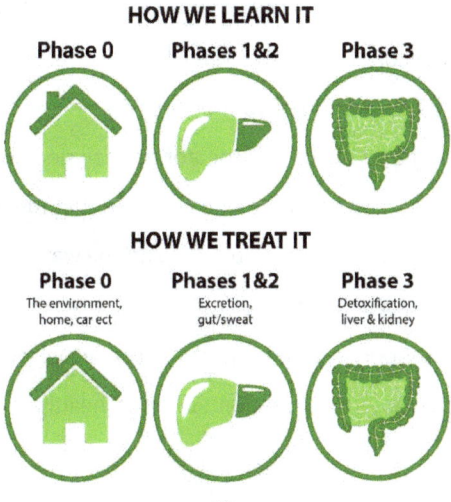

The 4 phases of detoxification are named phases 0, 1, 2 & 3 detoxification and each stage prepares the toxicant and uses specific enzymes and nutrients. These phases work together and are designed to protect and heal us. By supporting each phase individually, their synergistic activity is enhanced.

To confuse things a bit, although we will normally learn about detoxification in the order 0, 1, 2, and 3, it is better to treat in the opposite direction. Always address phase 0 (removing the source) first! So, after the source of exposure is removed, remember to assess gut health and the ability to sweat (Phase 3), then support phase 2 and 1! This is the order I will be introducing you the phases in the book.

When we are exposed to bad stuff like mould or heavy metals, our well-designed detox systems turn up the volume and work to make those substances less toxic and clear them out through bile, urine, and sweat predominantly. In times of overexposure, like in a source of water contamination or proximity to a large exposure source, our detox capabilities are outweighed by the toxic load. Remember the glass?

One thing to remember about finding out someone has a toxic burden, is that the severity of symptoms can help dictate how quickly you need to find and eliminate the sources of exposure. The more severe the symptoms, the higher the priority. Removing or rehabilitating the offending exposure is always necessary for full resolution and improved detoxification.

Step 1 - Assess and support Phase 0 - Remove the source, you cannot heal in the same environment that made you sick.

Every other phase is secondary to this one! Phase 0 refers to exposure, specifically, identifying it to remove it. You can check your environments using ERMI testing, agar plates or professional air sampling by a building inspector or analysing your water. Another part of this step is to eat clean, drink clean and breathe clean. So that means sourcing good quality food, filtering your water (both the water you drink and the water you bathe in), and filtering your air with a hepa/carbon air purifier.

If you don't remove the source of the bad stuff, it is virtually impossible to support the next 3 phases enough to remove it to the point of good health.

The first step in this phase would be the investigation stage, finding what the environmental toxin is and what the most likely sources are. This step is crucial to the full resolution of symptoms. Too many people want to get rid of their toxic burden from their body before determining the source. Unfortunately, it's almost impossible to detox while still in current exposure, remember, you cannot heal in the same environment that made you sick.

Most people don't know they have been or are being exposed to something harmful. I would have to say that it is highly unlikely that you even know that you have even been exposed! The sheer number of patients I have had, who claim there is no mould in their environment, who I have then asked to fully inspect for mould, and they have found it under the bed, behind a bookshelf, around a windowsill, in the ceiling or walls or even in the air-conditioning system of their car, is astounding!!! We are, in most cases, also not aware of the metals and persistent organic pollutants in our air, water, or food. Trying to pinpoint the actual past exposure can be both frustrating and unnecessary. It is better to understand where the ongoing or potential source of the next exposure is than to dwell on past exposures. Once you know the toxin or toxins that you are burdened with, finding and eliminating (or at the very least reducing the exposure) the most probable source of exposure is the top priority.

The next step, once you have established the potential source of the exposure, is to remove or rehabilitate it. This can be done by moving away from the source, rehabilitating the environment, or if neither of these is possible, the use of air and water purifiers can help

The source is usually within the environments you exist in. Your neighbourhood, your home, your office/school, and your car, and all can be the main sources and should all be investigated. Once you have done this, you can move on to supporting phases 3, 2 and 1 of detoxification in that order.

Something to consider before moving on to the 3 phases is whether you can physically handle detoxification. As discussed in the previous chapter, sometimes a little prep work before an active detox can make the process much more bearable!

Step 2 - Treat/support Phase 3 elimination (into the toilet or out the skin!):

Once toxic substances are sent through the liver to be bio-transformed and conjugated (a fancy way of saying 'packaged"), they must be eliminated. Phase 3 is the elimination stage of detox. Without proper support of elimination, toxins and potentially more toxic bio-transformed products will stay in the body longer.

Phase 3 is all about the gut, kidneys, and skin, but mostly the gut. Gut health is very important for proper detoxification. If you have too many bad bugs in your gut, they can create an enzyme called beta-glucuronidase. This enzyme takes the nicely packaged toxins and unwraps them. They are then reabsorbed into the bloodstream and need to go through phases 1 and 2 all over again! Please remember that gut detoxification should happen prior to liver detoxification. Moving toxins out of the liver and into a sluggish bowel can create autointoxication and, frankly, a very cranky person with hangover-type symptoms.

You can test for beta-glucuronidase using a poop test. But ideally you should assess the whole microbiome and gut health not just this enzyme. If you test above the reference range, there are things you can use to lower the enzyme activity. Saccharomyces boulardi, a probiotic yeast, can reduce bacterial species that produce beta-glucuronidase. S. boulardii is a great addition to most programs. Please make sure you aren't allergic to yeast before using it though.

Another supplement choice is calcium-D-glucarate. This compound can suppress blood and tissue beta-glucuronidase activity. It works to inhibit beta-glucuronidase activity in the liver, kidney, and intestinal microbiome tissue. Glucomannan fibre is also an excellent tool for lowering beta-glucuronidase.

Healthy bowel movements and healthy kidneys and urine are how we eliminate most toxins. If you suffer from urinary retention or constipation, up regulating the body's detox capacity would lead to the retention of and potential reabsorption of the bad things you are trying so hard to remove. If you are dehydrated or have any form of kidney damage, the kidneys will struggle to adequately filter and release toxins.

Many toxins are fat-soluble and get packed into bile to travel through the guts, but about 95 percent of bile is reabsorbed and recycled, along with many of the fat-soluble toxins. During detoxification, the reabsorption of the toxins from the gut back into the liver can impede healing as the toxin can be recirculated repeatedly before it's a part of the 5% of bile that gets excreted. To combat this recirculation phenomenon, binding agents are used. They act like static clings and attract specific compounds to them. The adsorbent nature of these compounds attracts bile and toxins and binds them tightly. Binders are a crucial piece to many treatment programs, whether they include removing environmental toxins, reducing toxin exposure, or treating infections. Binders can be eaten, or taken orally in pill, powder, gel, or tincture form. Different binders can attract different toxins, so knowing which one to use can make or break a protocol. Some common binders include:

Zeolite:

Zeolite is formed from volcanic rock and ash and is a well-known binder for heavy metals and other toxins.

Clay:

Bentonite and zeolite clays have been touted as working wonders in the cosmetic industry and are also commonly used as binding agents for detoxification.

Activated Charcoal:

Activated charcoal is a fine black powder made from bone char, coconut shells, peat, petroleum coke, coal, olive pits, or sawdust.

Chlorella:

Chlorella is a type of freshwater algae that is rich in chlorophyll and is known to bind to heavy metals and other toxins.

Modified Citrus Pectin:

Modified citrus pectin is a soluble fibre derived from the pulp and peels of citrus fruits that has been modified to make it easier for the body to absorb.

Unfortunately, Bile can be released from the binding agent if left too long in the gut without moving into the toilet. In the intestines, there are also bad bug enzymes that can break down some glucuronide and sulphide bonds and cause resorption of toxic compounds. This is why constipation is the enemy and ensuring adequate bowel movements prior to adding detox factors and binders is an important top priority. By priming Phase 3 detox, all the wonderful work done to support Phases 1 and 2 will mean that toxins will be easily eliminated and flushed away.

If you become constipated, you can use magnesium citrate or magnesium oxide to assist in bowel movements. You can dose up until you are having comfortable daily bowel movements. If things run smoothly, then toxins come into the body and are swiftly removed into the toilet.

Step 3 - treat/support Phases 2 and 1 - packaging the bad stuff to make it harmless and easy to excrete:

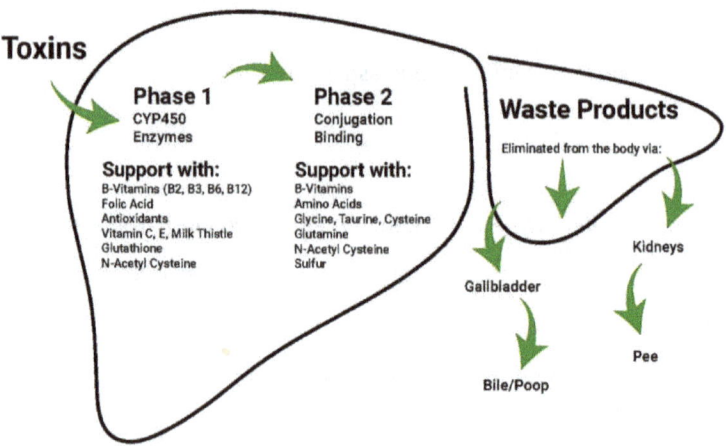

Phase 2 detoxification is the second step in the body's detoxification process. It is also known as the conjugation pathway, where the liver attaches another molecule to the "intermediate toxin" to render it harmless and ready for the toilet. It involves enzymes which are made from specific genes. The genes will be discussed in detail later in the book.

For the rest of this chapter I will cover the Phase 2 pathways, touch on the enzymes and then dive deeper into those enzymes in the next chapter.

An overview of the six types of conjugation pathways that take place in Phase 2:

Sulphation: This pathway uses sulphur-containing compounds, mostly from stinky vegetables like broccoli and cabbage, to neutralise toxins

Glucuronidation: This pathway uses glucuronic acid to neutralise toxins. Glucuronic acid is a type of sugar that helps remove harmful substances from the body. Glucuronic acid binds to the bad stuff in the liver and then this package is passed in the urine. This is the main pathway most mycotoxins are packaged by. There are a few foods listed later in the chapter than can support this pathway.

Glutathione conjugation: This pathway uses glutathione to neutralise toxins. It is VERY important to support glutathione through supplementing NAC, Glycine, reduced or liposomal glutathione and by eating stinky vegetables.

Methylation: This pathway binds a methyl groups (a carbon and three hydrogens) to a variety of toxins. It needs magnesium and the B vitamins. You can eat liver, leafy greens and beets to support this pathway.

Acetylation: This pathway uses acetyl groups to neutralise toxins. You can support this by supplementing vitamin C and eating a mediterranean diet.

Glycination: This pathway uses the amino acid glycine to neutralise toxins. You can support this by supplementing glycine or eating foods rich in glycine.

Sulphation:

The sulphation pathway is dependent on inorganic sulphate molecules found in protein, stinky vegetables (cruciferous and allium vegetables) and some supplements and is important in the detoxification of the following substances:

Oestrogen

Progesterone

DHEA

Melatonin

Triiodothyronine (T3)

Tetraiodothyronine (T4)

Dopamine

Adrenaline/Epinephrine

Norepinephrine

Bisphenol A (BPA)

Triclosan Benoxophenone-3

Butylated Hydroxytoluene (BHT)

BPA which is found in plastics, liners of food and drink cans, liners of water pipes, plastic cling wraps, lacquers, varnishes, inks, adhesives, flame retardants, dental sealants & composite materials, sunglasses, water coolers, sports equipment and thermal receipts, like the ones you get every time you buy something.

Triclosan, an antibacterial found in cleaning and personal care products; also used in kitchenware, computer equipment, clothes, and children's toys.

Benoxophenone-3 which is found in sunscreens, nail polish, makeup, hair & skin care.

Butylated Hydroxytoluene (BHT) a food additive/preservative in butter, meats, cereals, chewing gum, baked goods, snack foods, and dehydrated potatoes, and is also used in animal feed, cosmetics, pharmaceuticals, rubber, petroleum, and electrical transformers.

There are several reasons why someone may not have sufficient sulphate levels or have an impaired ability to conjugate sulphate. These include a low protein diet, low intake of sulphate-rich foods, high toxin exposure (which depletes sulphate), low magnesium levels, and issues with the sulfotransferase (SULTs) family of enzymes.

Nutrients that support Sulphation:

Eating more sulphur-containing amino acids (cysteine, methionine, and taurine) can help.

Cruciferous vegetables (broccoli, cauliflower, cabbage, brussels sprouts, kale etc.),

Allium vegetables (onions, garlics, leeks, shallots, chives)

Eggs or protein in general

Other things that can help are NAC or glutathione.

Epsom Salt (Magnesium Sulphate) Baths are a great way to increase sulphation in someone who doesn't tolerate sulphate-rich foods in the diet.

Going out into the sun stimulates the production of cholesterol sulphate.

Glucuronidation:

Glucuronidation is the process of adding glucuronic acid to a toxic byproduct to make it water-soluble. This is one of the most prevalent in drug metabolism but especially important for the detoxification of mycotoxins.

This pathway is also important for the metabolism of hormones, bilirubin, and some medications as listed:

Plastics
Oestrogens
Androgens (Testosterone, DHEA)
Thyroid hormones (T3 &T4)
Bilirubin
Some (most) Mycotoxins
And some medications.

It is estimated that up to 40-70% of all medications are metabolised by glucuronidation. Examples include:

- NSAID's
- Benzodiazepines (Lorazepam)
- Tylenol (Paracetamol)
- Codeine
- Morphine

Nutrients that support Glucuronidation:

Resveratrol	Dandelion
Curcumin	Rooibos tea
D-limonene	Honeybush tea
Quercetin	Rosemary
Citrus Fruits	Astaxanthin
Cruciferous vegetables	Calcium-d-glucurate

Glutathione conjugation:

This pathway is by far the most important pathway for many of the environmental toxins and carcinogens we are exposed to daily. This process uses the enzyme glutathione-S-transferase (GST), and is dependent on glutathione, which is a tripeptide comprised of cysteine, glutamine, and glycine.

Glutathione is the body's chief antioxidant, and its actions within the detoxification pathways are multifaceted. This is why glutathione is one of the TOP supplements recommended for detoxification.

Glutathione conjugation occurs in phase 2 detoxification for the following elements:

Pesticides and herbicides
Heavy metals, especially:
- Mercury
- Lead
- Arsenic
- Cadmium
Most Mycotoxins
Some medications:
- Tylenol (Acetaminophen)
- Alcohol
- Tetracycline

The main factor that impairs glutathione conjugation is glutathione deficiency. Many chronic illnesses are associated with glutathione deficiency, and this is believed to be due to increased utilisation to combat oxidative stress and overall toxic burden. This means, we are using more than we can make due to the increasing need from our toxic exposures!

By adding in NAC and Glycine, the precursors, or glutathione supplementation, this common Phase 2 enzymatic reaction can be readily supported. If you are going to supplement glutathione, be aware that only certain forms are well absorbed, such as the S-Acetyl-glutathione or Liposomal Glutathione.

Foods and nutrients will also support the glutathione S-transferase enzymes:

Garlic	Rooibos tea
Fish oil	Honeybush tea
Black soybean	Ellagic acid

Purple sweet potato	Rosemary
Curcumin	Ghee
Green tea	Genistein

Glutathione needs to be reduced, acetylated or liposomal. You can add NAC and Glycine to help endogenous Glutathione production. Glutathione recyclers include Vitamin C, Vitamin E. Because glutathione is a master antioxidant as well as being involved in detoxification, it is important to reduce free radicals to prevent glutathione depletion. Omega 3 supplementation, alpha lipoic acid, and selenium can all help.

Increase the stinky, cruciferous vegetables (rich in sulphur) and protein (for ample amounts of cysteine, glycine, and glutamine).

You can assess oxidative stress and glutathione needs in blood by assessing blood markers:

1 - Gamma-glutamyl Transferase (GGT) - GGT is a marker for glutathione depletion in the liver, and elevations in GGT reflect increased need for support. Curcumin, an Indian spice found in turmeric and curry powder, has been shown to improve elevated GGT. Liposomal glutathione, reduced glutathione, S-acetyl glutathione, NAC and Glycine also help.

2 - Uric acid - This is usually associated with gout and arthritis. However, recently, it has come to light that levels above 7mg/dL in the blood also imply severe oxidative stress, which can lead to glutathione depletion. The goal would be to get this number to 5 mg/dL using diet and supplements where indicated. Uric acid is increased in diets that are high in glucose and fructose, as well as excess sodium chloride, so reducing those can help significantly, as well as reducing alcohol and organ meats, as well as some fish and seafood. Vitamin C, quercetin, and tart cherries have been shown to reduce uric acid levels, and this reduces glutathione depletion.

3 - Bilirubin - For decades, bilirubin has been believed to be a toxic waste product of haem catabolism in humans, while in recent years, accumulating evidence has shown that bilirubin has beneficial effects on various oxidative stress-associated diseases.

4 - Albumin - It has been showing that albumin is involved in many bioactive functions such as regulation of plasma osmotic pressure, binding and transport of various endogenous

or exogenous compounds, but most people don't know that it is also a powerful antioxidant used for extracellular antioxidant defences. Low Albumin is indicative of oxidative stress and should be supported with the appropriate diet and supplements.

You can also assess oxidative stress using urinary 8-Hydroxy-2'-deoxyguanosine (8-OHdG). This is a marker of DNA damage from oxidative stress, and high levels immediately infer a higher need for all antioxidants, not just glutathione. There are also urinary organic acid markers that can indicate a higher need for Glutathione. Specifically, Pyroglutamic Acid and 2-Hydroxybutyric Acid, which can be seen in an organic acid urine test.

Methylation:

Methylation is central to such critical reactions in the body as:

- Repairing and building RNA and DNA
- Immune function (how your body responds to and fights infection)
- Digestive issues
- DNA silencing
- Neurotransmitter balance
- Metal Detoxification
- Inflammation
- Membrane fluidity
- Energy production
- Protein activity
- Myelination
- Cancer prevention

Methylation is involved in many biochemical processes throughout the body, so it is no surprise that it is also involved in detoxification. In detoxification, a methyl group (CH3) is added to toxins to make them water-soluble. This process uses a family of enzymes called methyl transferases. One of the most famous of these enzymes is catechol-O-methyltransferase (COMT), which it's known for its role in metabolising oestrogens and neurotransmitters like adrenaline and dopamine. You can assess the activity of COMT, including the potential for it to be too fast or too slow thanks to genetics, through a variety of tests. Although more commonly recognised as a methylation enzyme, MTHFR is not the most common issue when it comes to methylation but should be assessed in relation to COMT. There is a hole chapter dedicated to methylation, so you are going to get more information later!

Methylation is used to detox the following:

Oestrogen
Adrenaline/Epinephrine
Noradrenaline/Norepinephrine
Dopamine
Histamine
Arsenic
Phenols

Phenols can be found in coal tar, petroleum, plastics, vaccine preservatives, and Botox. Aromatic hydrocarbons are carcinogens found in cigarette smoke, dyes, adhesives, perfume, pharmaceuticals, pesticides, explosives, diesel exhaust, combustion of wood chips, and grilled meats and fish.

Methylation can be impaired in several ways, such as stress, toxin exposure, and more! While methylation genes can be part of the picture, they are by no means close to the full picture. Methylation genes tell us genetic predisposition but do not tell us phenotypic expression, which can be influenced by nutrient levels, gut health, toxic load, and use of methylation inhibitors (such as birth control pills, PPI's, antibiotics, nitrous oxide, valproic acid, and cholestyramine). Additionally, other factors, such as sucrose (sugar), have been found to slow down methylation enzymes.

Look for signs of low methylation, including histamine issues (where you get red and itchy), elevated homocysteine, MCH, and MCV (the size and health of red blood cells), low red blood cell folate, and low serum B12. Measuring homocysteine can be used to support the dosing of methylation factors to support detoxification. But it's not the only way to assess the process, there are way more complex tests that look at the whole process, but these would need to be prescribed by your practitioner.

You can also assess elevated urinary Methylmalonic Acid or MMA (Vitamin B12) and Formiminoglutamic acid or FIGLU (Folate) as organic acid markers in the urine.

Methylation is supported by cofactors and methyl donors like folate, methionine, B2, vitamin B12, vitamin B6, betaine, folate, and magnesium. Food high in protein will provide methionine, and legumes, seeds, liver, leaf greens, avocado, asparagus, and certain grains can provide food sources of other vitamins and nutrients.

Acetylation:

The process of acetylation attaches a molecule called an acetyl Co-A molecule to the toxin to make it less harmful.

Acetylation is responsible for the metabolism of the following types of toxins:

Caffeine
Benzodiazepines
Noradrenaline/Norepinephrine
Isoniazid
Hydralazine
Sulphonamides
Histamine
Aromatic amines

Aromatic amines are carcinogens found in cigarette smoke, dyes, adhesives, perfume, pharmaceuticals, pesticides, explosives diesel exhaust, combustion of wood chips, and grilled meats and fish.

Glycination:

There are several types of amino acid conjugation (binding) reactions that occur in phase 2 detoxification. Glycination is the most common type of amino acid conjugation and is mostly used when detoxing salicylates and benzoates. Benzoate is widely used in food preservatives, while salicylates can be found naturally in our food supply and in synthetic forms within medications and personal care products. This pathway is dependent on enough of the amino acid glycine. To support glycination you need to decrease the intake of salicylates and benzoates.

Glycination is responsible for the metabolism of the following types of toxins:

Non-food salicylates:
Aspirin and 5-SA compounds similar to aspirin
Alka Seltzer
Various non-steroidal anti-inflammatory drugs

Food salicylates:
Fruits: apricots, blackberries, blueberries, cantaloupe, cherries, cranberry, currants, dates, grapes, guava, loganberries, orange, pineapple, plums, prunes, raisins, raspberries, strawberries.
Vegetables: capsicum, chili, mushroom, olives, pepper (sweet), radish, tomato, zucchini.
Seeds/Nuts: almonds, peanuts.

Spices: anise, cayenne, celery, cinnamon, cumin, curry powder, dill, fenugreek, five spice, ginger, honey, mint, mustard, oregano, rosemary, sage, turmeric, thyme.

Food Dyes:
Salicylic acid is also found in some personal care products such as fragrances and perfumes, cosmetics, toothpaste, mouthwash, muscle pain creams, sunscreens, and skin care products. Toluene is a popular industrial chemical that is converted into benzoate within the liver. It can be found in homes with paint thinners, paint brush cleaners, nail polish, glues, inks, and stain removers.

Sodium Benzoate is a widely used preservative in food, medications, and personal care products. There is some concern that sodium benzoate can convert into the carcinogenic molecule benzene - this has been shown to happen on soda and other products that also contain vitamin C. Additional concerns also exist around increased risk for hyperactivity behaviour.

Foods that can help as they are high in high in glycine:

Almonds	Lobster
Amaranth	Most fish
Beef	Mung beans
Chicken	Pork

Collagen protein	Pumpkin seeds
Duck	Seaweed
Eggs	Soybeans
Goose	Sunflower seeds
Lamb	Turkey
Lentils	

Amino acid conjugation:

Amino acid conjugation involves the binding of toxic carboxylic acids, bile acids, and xenobiotics to the amino group of amino acids. The most common amino acids used are aspartate and glutamate. Other amino acids used are taurine, glycine, lysine, serine, proline, ornithine, glutamine, and valine. A protein-rich diet will supply these amino acids.

The family of enzymes involved in acetylation are supported with a protein-rich diet, choline, vitamin D, vitamin B12, and quercetin. Vitamin B1, Vitamin B5, and Vitamin C can also help.

That concludes Phase 2!

The original toxins are now water soluble and are deposited into bile or sent to the kidneys, ready to be eliminated via phase 3 detoxification. Assessing Phase 0 and then Supporting Phase II detoxification can be a powerful tool in achieving optimal results in detoxification.

Phase 1 - making things worse before they get better

Phase 1 detoxification is the first step in breaking toxins down and transforming harmful substances into less harmful water-soluble molecules that can be eliminated from the body. Unfortunately, the toxins can become even more toxic at this stage, producing products called free radicals, also known as reactive oxygen species, that can inflame and oxidise healthy cells! And we don't want that!

These intermediary toxins are then acted upon in Phase 2 for conjugation (getting safely bound to something like an amino acid) and excretion. Due to the dose-dependent and time-dependent nature of toxin exposure, if exposure rates outweigh the body's detox capability, some of these Phase 1 bio-transformed compounds can build up if not immediately conjugated (safely bond up for excretion) by Phase 2 in a timely manner. If Phase 1 is faster than Phase 2, this is often when individuals suffer from symptoms prior to Phase 2 supportive therapies. To support the effects of Phase 1, we support the Phase 2 enzyme functions through nutrition and lifestyle. This will assist in the conversion and eventual safe clearance of the toxins into the toilet and is all why we treat phase 3 before 2 and 1!

I won't talk too much about this phase because, in practice, addressing phases 0, 2, and 3 will give you the results you are looking for! All that you need to take home from this phase is that it can make more bad stuff if phases 2 and 3 are not optimal!

There are four main challenges when detoxing.

First, excessive exposure to toxins will obviously overtax the system.

Second, either or both Phase 2 and 3 can be slow.

Third, if Phase 1 is fast or Phase 2 is slow, intermediary metabolites will build up. The intermediary substances are highly reactive.

Finally, if both are slow, substances are not being detoxed properly at a proper speed, resulting in further accumulation. Clinically, this is the very sick, sensitive-to-everything patient who will require an extra measure of patience and time.

These challenges can all be met if you follow the advice to treat in the order of Phase 0, 3 2 and 1.

The other detox systems

Other systems that need to be supported are sweating and the lymphatic system. You can sweat through exercise or the use of an infra-red sauna.

Lymph drainage is important in detoxification because it promotes and improves the function of the lymphatic system. The lymphatic system is a vital part of the body's immune defence and waste elimination system. It collects excess tissue fluid and transports it back to the bloodstream. It also absorbs nutrients from the digestive system and transports waste products. When functioning properly, it removes dead virus and bacteria cells from the tissues, reduces excess fluid, and promotes blood cell replenishment.

Unlike the cardiovascular system that has a heart to pump the blood around, the lymphatic fluid relies on your skeletal muscles contracting and relaxing through exercise in order to move the lymph fluid. Lymphatic drainage massage is a gentle massage technique that can help to move the lymph. Other things that can help gently move your lymph are rebounding on a small trampoline and dry skin brushing.

Using herbs is a popular way to naturally purify your lymphatic system. Calendula, echinacea, and dandelion are just a few of the many herbs that promote lymphatic drainage, reduce any swelling and pain, and boost your immune system. Drinking water is crucial to every aspect of your health, including your lymph system. Drinking at least eight glasses of water a day will keep fluids moving through your lymphatic system.

As you can see, there are various factors that determine the rate by which toxins and toxicants accumulate in the body. For instance, genetics, occupation, lifestyle, work, and home environments are often missed or not asked about in a medical assessment.

Diet and lifestyle play a major role in whether you will remove the bad stuff or not. Proper nutrition and consistent ingestion of helpful detoxification nutrients or phytonutrients can impact your body's ability to adequately reduce the presence of toxicants and lower the body's burden. There are recipes and a Reset program on the website to help support your process.

A little tip:

Perhaps the most difficult part of working with patients through detox is patient compliance. A significant portion of our position is to teach, inspire and motivate our patients. You can give choices to the patient as long as they understand the ramifications of their choice. Strongly recommend the best choice to fit the patient, not necessarily the one you think they want to hear. Explain the process to them so they understand that there will be times they feel better and times when they may feel 'worse while they improve. Be there for them as they go through the process, and if you can't be there, get a coach to help them.

If you are a patient reading this, then the sentiment in the previous paragraph is that YOU are in control of your health outcomes, not your doctor, your nutritionist, or your coach. So, YOU need to be compliant, make the changes, and put in the work so that YOU can achieve optimal health!

Chapter 9: The Basics of Genes and Enzymes

I remember the day I learned that we could control the outcomes of our genes through diet and lifestyle. That day changed my life! Which is why I want to introduce you to some basics about genetics and hopefully inspire you to change the outcome of yours. You can't change the genes you are born with, not unless you are bitten by a radioactive spider (like spiderman was) or have a bone marrow transplant, but you can change whether they work well or not. That is called "gene expression".

During gene expression, the DNA is read and then turned into a protein, such as an enzyme, that performs a function. These enzymes are important for keeping us healthy by doing many things in the body, but also for removing bad things so we can heal. Essentially, genes are codes for enzymes that can help us function better, however; sometimes they don't function as well as they should due to an error in spelling as described below. The good news is, that the outcomes or expression of all the genes I will discuss later, can all be improved through some changes in diet, lifestyle, stress management, better sleep or supplements!

I like to think of genes as the "words" in the "Book of Life." These words join up to make sentences that can eventually be read as your life story. Each gene is made up of 2 nucleotides made from the letters A, G, T and C. One that you inherited from your mom and another that you inherited from your dad. The problem with genes is that some of them have 'spelling errors" called single nucleotide polymorphisms or SNPs, and some (not all) of these SNP's can affect how well the enzymes will function in the body.

There are thousands of SNPs, but not all of them are important when it comes to health. There are a few that have risen to the top of the pile of importance by being relevant to health but also by being actionable, which means you have some degree of control over whether a mutation or SNP is indeed a good or a bad thing to have.

Many of us have these common SNP's that make it more difficult for us to process and remove certain toxins from our bodies. SNP research has shown that one person compared to another, may have anywhere between a 2x to 10x faster or slower clearance of certain toxicants. Thankfully we can now test and support these genes to help us become healthier and less toxic. As an example, that people can relate to, I often refer to SNPs as words that can be read and interpreted according to the spelling. If we take the word Gray and the word Grey. They are spelled slightly differently, but if used in the sentence "I need a grey/gray coat," you would most likely think that the person needed a coat that was the colour grey. If, however, they needed a coat, but the word was spelled goat - that would result in a very different outcome!

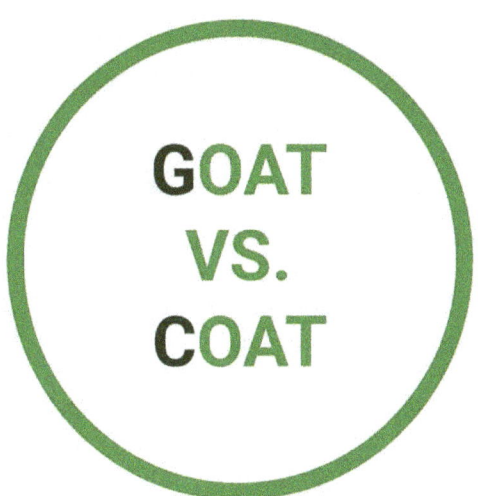

Genes make enzymes which are proteins that act as biological catalysts. Catalysts accelerate chemical reactions. The molecules upon which enzymes may act are called substrates, and the enzyme converts the substrates into different molecules known as metabolites. Luckily, both the genes and the metabolites can be tested. To test genes, we need a cheek swab or some saliva or blood. For the metabolites we can check using a simple urine test, so we can determine which enzyme needs extra support!

If you run a genetic test, always make sure that the test looks for the specific gene that is well-researched and is actionable through diet, lifestyle, or nutrition. There is no point in testing every gene in the body as not all affect health, and not all are actionable.

Most importantly is that you cover genes that affect inflammation, detoxification, and oxidative stress. There are also some that infer a higher need for certain nutrients like Vitamin A and D, or essential fats. Those can be useful for overall health as well.

When assessing genetic predispositions, I recommend assessing organ systems rather than a single gene. Although there are MANY genes you could assess, I am going to focus on just a few that would help! Your service provider may have information on other relevant genes as it is a HUGE topic, but if you cover the basics, you should be OK when removing toxins.

When it comes to toxins, the following should be assessed, please note there are many more genes that CAN be assessed, these are some of the basics, also the abbreviations listed are to make it easier to read the enzyme names, the full names will be provided in the next chapter: Note that the codes you see below, are actually abbreviations of the enzyme name!

Phase 1 - CYP (Cytochrome P450) genes - there are a lot, but a few are most relevant

Methylation - MTHFD1, MTHFR, MTR, MTRR, COMT, CBS

Detoxification - CYP, GST, NQ01, SULT

Inflammation - IL6, TNF-alpha, and the other small IL genes

Oxidative stress - eNOS, MnSOD, CAT, GPX1

Nutritional needs - VDR, CYP2R1, GC, FADS, BCO1, FUT2, GSTT1, HLA for gluten sensitivity and MCM6 for dairy intolerance.

Over the next few chapters I will cover the genes and enzymes of the biological systems that affect or are affected by exposure to environmental toxins, lifestyle, stress, nutrition and sleep and help you action on any that you may find you have!

Chapter 10: Methylation Genes

Methylation is a biochemical process that controls the body's ability to detox and lower inflammation, produce neurotransmitters, and protect DNA. Methylation depends on several vitamins and cofactors, including choline, magnesium, folate, vitamin B12, and vitamin B6. Deficiency in these critical vitamins can be caused by a poor diet, genetic mutations, toxic exposure, high stress, virus, infection, or any combination of these. Methylation is relevant to life and health, from early development to immunity, memory formation, and more. Impaired methylation can lead to conditions like depression, anxiety, histamine intolerance, hormonal imbalance, poor detox ability, birth defects, increased risk for cancer, fatigue, and low energy.

Methylation, also commonly termed "one-carbon metabolism," is a biochemical process that involves the transfer of active methyl groups. Methyl groups consist of a hydrogen attached to three carbons (-CH3) and can be formed in two ways:

1. By adding a hydrogen molecule ("reduction") to methylene (-CH2-) groups, by the enzyme methylene tetra hydro folate reductase (MTHFR).

2. By the transfer of a complete methyl group, such as is done by catechol-O-methyltransferase (COMT). Methyltransferase enzymes use methyl groups donated from the universal active methyl transfer compound S-adenosylmethionine (SAMe).

Let's have a look at some of the genes involved in methylation, on reading the full name, you will realise why we abbreviate them:

Methylenetetrahydrofolate dehydrogenase 1 (MTHFD1) gene: The MTHFD1 gene is involved in producing biologically active folate and may increase requirements for choline. Choline, an essential nutrient, plays a central role in many physiological pathways in the body, including homocysteine metabolism, neurotransmitter synthesis, cell-membrane signalling, and transport of bile and lipoproteins and is vital during a mycotoxin detox. Requirements for choline vary based on gender (post-menopausal women need more regardless of genetics), age, physical activity level as well as genetics. If you test and find you have an SNP in MTHFD1, increase your intake of choline-rich foods such as eggs, beef and beef liver, and salmon. Supplementation would be advised where requirements exceed dietary intake, such as in post-menopausal women or mould exposure. Also, ensure adequate intake of betaine-rich foods like beets, broccoli, leafy greens, and seafood and avoid folate deficiency.

Methylenetetrahydrofolate Reductase (MTHFR) gene - MTHFR is a key enzyme in the folate metabolism pathway – directing folate from the diet either to DNA synthesis or homocysteine re-methylation. The MTHFR enzyme is the rate-limiting step of the methylation cycle, and decreased MTHFR activity can greatly impact downstream reactions as well as contribute to the build-up of potentially harmful molecules, such as homocysteine. It is estimated that up to 85% of the general population has at least 1 MTHFR SNP variant that impacts this methylation process.

It is a low penetrance gene, which means the even though the SNP is common, the impact of the SNP is lower than previously thought. The SNP can thankfully be easily addressed through a healthy, folate-rich diet as well as nutritional supplements like B2 or folate (although some people can react to methylated supplements, so please get professional advice before supplementing), as well as lifestyle adjustments like stress management and toxin avoidance.

If you have an SNP in MTHFR, please don't assume the worst and start taking ALL the methyl donor supplements, I have seen this happen, and unfortunately, methylation is a balancing act where you can either be under-methylating and NEED nutritional support or over-methylating, which means certain supplements can cause or worsen different complications like anxiety. This can be remedied with low-dose Niacin (B3), but it's better to avoid getting there in the first place!

The next two genes act together; they are MTR and MTRR - SNPs in the MTR and MTRR genes can affect methylation in several ways. Here are some key points:

Methionine synthase (MTR), Methionine synthase reductase (MTRR) genes: SNPs in the MTRR gene impair MTR activity, resulting in elevated homocysteine levels due to compromised methylation to methionine. MTRR requires vitamin B12 and folate to function optimally.

The MTR gene and its linked B12 deficiency risk has been associated with various health outcomes, including neural tube defects and spina bifida.

SNPs in the MTR and MTRR genes can affect methylation due to the high risk of B12 deficiencies in people with the SNP impairing MTR activity, leading to elevated homocysteine levels and abnormal DNA methylation. If you have SNP's in either of these two genes, please make sure you get adequate amounts of B12 through diet or supplements and reduce alcohol intake as it is a known inhibitor of these enzymes.

Catechol-O-methyltransferase (COMT) gene: The COMT gene is responsible for making an enzyme called catechol-O-methyltransferase, which helps to detox hormones like oestrogen and catecholamines neurotransmitters like dopamine,

norepinephrine/noradrenaline, and epinephrine/adrenaline, as well as drugs and substances that have the same catechol structure as these biological substances.

Magnesium is an important mineral for the activity of COMT. SNP's in COMT tend to slow this enzyme down. If the enzyme is slow, it can be assisted with Magnesium supplements. There are also a few nutrients that can further slow the enzyme down. These include green tea and quercetin, so please do get assessed before assuming you can safely take certain supplements!

Because COMT is a methylation gene, it's essential to get adequate B vitamins to support COMT, especially B2, B6, B9, and B12, along with magnesium.

If you have a SNP in COMT that slows it down, eat more stinky vegetables like broccoli and cauliflower, eat your onions, and make sure you get enough magnesium into you.

People who don't have a SNP in COMT (meaning it is faster not slower), need to drink green tea and learn to love life more.

In either case, reduce your toxic exposure!

Signs that you are under-methylating:

High histamine and inflammatory markers can indicate under methylation, as can a mild increase of homocysteine in the blood (hyperhomocysteinemia). This can be a risk factor for a variety of common conditions, including high blood pressure, blood clots, pregnancy loss, psychiatric disorders, and certain types of cancer. Folate deficiency can cause macrocytosis, which is an increase in the mean corpuscular volume (MCV), or overall size of red blood cells as less mature red blood cells are released into the bloodstream.

MTHFR SNPs in women can affect a woman's egg quality and increase the risk of neural tube defects, miscarriages, and pregnancy complications. This is why it is so important to assess before pregnancy.

Signs that you are over-methylating
(usually from taking the wrong supplements):

Anxiety: Individuals who are over methylated may experience high levels of anxiety.

Depression: Over methylation can be associated with symptoms of depression.

Panic Attacks: People who are over methylated may be more prone to experiencing panic attacks.

Hyperactivity: Over methylation can manifest as hyperactivity or restlessness.

Poor Concentration: Difficulty concentrating or focusing may be a symptom of over methylation.

Sleep Disorders: Over methylation can contribute to sleep disturbances, such as insomnia or restless sleep.

Histamine Intolerance: Over methylation may be associated with sensitivities to foods and chemicals, as well as histamine intolerance.

High Pain Threshold: Individuals who are over methylated may have a higher pain threshold.

Elevated Neurotransmitter Levels: Over methylation can lead to elevated levels of neurotransmitters like dopamine, norepinephrine, and serotonin.

Summary of Methylation SNPS, if you have a SNP here's what you can do:

MTHFD1 - Increase Choline

MTHFR - Increase B vitamins, especially B2 and folate

MTR & MTRR - B12 need may be higher

COMT slow - Increase Magnesium and B vitamins

COMT fast - Green tea & Quercetin

Chapter 11: Detoxification Genes

It is important to note that detoxification is a complex process that is influenced by many factors, not just genetics. Other factors that can influence detoxification are your environment and lifestyle. Assessing the genes is just one piece of the detoxification puzzle. It is also important not to treat genetic results as a diagnosis of disease. The genes discussed below are all actionable! They are like switches in the body that can be turned on or off with nutrients and lifestyle changes. They don't mean you are doomed to the consequences, just that they potentially need some additional support from you and your habits,

Phase I detoxification: This is carried out primarily through the family of Cytochrome P450 enzymes (there are a lot, and they all start with CYP).

The CYP450 superfamily of enzymes metabolises toxic compounds of exogenous (environmental toxins) or endogenous (like hormones made by our own body) origin in Phase I detoxification reactions. SNPs located within genes involved in Phase I detoxification can affect the activity of CYP450 enzymes.

To improve the outcome of anyone with significant CYP SNP's, you will need to ensure reduced exposure to the toxins (Support phase 0) as well improve Phase 2 and 3 detoxifications.

Phase 2 detoxification: As you noticed, phase 2 has 6 main pathways and each one has a variety of genes and enzymes associated with that pathway.

The glutathione transferases (GST) family of genes - These genes affect detoxification via glutathione conjugation by encoding for enzymes that play a key role in the detoxification of xenobiotics (things that aren't hormones but act like hormones), including some mycotoxins, heavy metals and BPA. They also protect cells against oxidative stress.

GSTs are typically small proteins that are activated in response to oxidative damage and/or exposure to a large variety of toxins. The GSTM1 enzyme helps the body detoxify several types of carcinogens, drugs, toxins, and oxidative stress.

Research suggests that consuming bitter herbs that promote liver health, such as milk thistle and dandelion, can support GST genes and Phase 2 detox. Other nutrients that can help are cruciferous vegetables such as broccoli, cabbage, brussels sprouts, as well as supplements such as N-Acetyl Cysteine and Glycine.

Quinone reductase (NQO1) gene - The gene NQO1 encodes a protein known as quinone reductase, which is a protein that plays a role in cellular protection and detoxification. Quinone reductase (QR) is an enzyme that plays an important role in the detoxification of quinones, which are highly reactive intermediates (created between phases 1 and 2 detox). Quinones are problematic as they can bind to and subsequently damage DNA and this can be a causing factor for some cancers!

NQO1 levels in cells can increase rapidly under stress conditions, especially those created by quinones. If you have a SNP in NQO1 you may benefit from Co-enzyme Q10 and Sulforaphane. Sulforaphane is a potent inducer of NQO1, meaning it improves the activity. Sulforaphane is a sulphur-rich compound found in many cruciferous vegetables like broccoli sprouts, cabbage, and cauliflower.

Heating broccoli may deactivate the enzyme that produces sulforaphane, but the process can be reactivated in cooked broccoli by chopping the broccoli at least 40 minutes before cooking or by adding a bit of mustard powder to the cooked broccoli. Sulforaphane supplements made from broccoli sprouts are also available, but whole-food sources are generally more effective.

Sulfotransferase 1A1 (SULT1A1) gene - SULT is involved in the inactivation of oestrogens and environmental toxins. SNP's carriers have a substantially lower activity of this enzyme.

Along with the addition of cruciferous or other sulphur-containing food like the album vegetables (onions, leeks and garlic) and supplements, people with a SNP in SULT should increase insoluble fibre, avoid refined carbohydrates.

Summary of Methylation SNPS, if you have a SNP here's what you can do:

CYP - support phases 2 and 3
GST - eat your stinky cruciferous vegetables
NQ01 - eat broccoli sprouts and take CoQ10
SULT - eat your stinky cruciferous and allium vegetables for the sulphur

Chapter 12: Inflammation Genes

Just like detoxification is a complex process, so is inflammation. Inflammation is a necessary step in the healing process if it is short lived and resolves the problem, however, some SNPs can predispose you to having chronic inflammation that doesn't resolve problems, it makes more problems! These SNP are again, actionable through diet and lifestyle. Gentle exercise and good sleep both help along with an anti-inflammatory diet.

Interleukin 6 (IL-6): IL-6 is a chemical messenger called a cytokine that is produced in the body wherever there is inflammation, either acute or chronic. It is involved in immune responses, inflammation and C-reactive protein (CRP) regulation, haematopoiesis (blood production), bone metabolism, and embryonic development.

This functional SNP has been associated with raised IL-6 and C-reactive protein or CRP (a blood marker that assess inflammation) concentrations and has been associated with inflammation, obesity, insulin resistance, dyslipidaemia, and raised blood pressure. All of these are generally worse in smokers.

Anyone with a SNP in this gene should follow a diet that reduces inflammation and includes increasing omega fatty acids, decreasing sources of trans fat from highly processed foods and replacing them with mono-unsaturated fats. Moderating omega six fatty acid intake from seeds and grains and increasing their intake of vegetables and antioxidant-rich foods. If dietary intake of omega fatty acids is inadequate, such as in a case where someone refuses to eat oily fish, supplementation may be required. A healthy weight and avoidance of all smoking are also imperative in managing inflammation.

Tumour necrosis factor-α (TNFα): TNFα is a pro-inflammatory cytokine secreted by both macrophages (white blood cells) and adipocytes (fat cells), that has been shown to alter whole-body glucose metabolism and has been implicated in the development of obesity, obesity-related insulin resistance, and issues with cholesterol.

If you have a SNP in this gene, you could improve your healthy by achieving and maintaining a healthy weight and fat percentage. Avoid smoking. Increase your intake of omega 3 fatty acids, reduce trans-fat intake. And just like with IL-6, if your dietary intake of omega 3 fatty acids is inadequate, supplementation may be required.

A high-sensitivity CRP (Hs-CRP) blood test may give further insight for at-risk individuals with either of these 2 SNP's.

Summary of the inflammation genes:

IL6 - increase Omega 3 in the form of fatty fish or supplements

TNF alpha - increase Omega 3 in the form of fatty fish or supplements

Chapter 13: Oxidative Stress Genes

Free radicals are a normal by-product of the body's energy-generating biochemical processes. They are highly reactive with other molecules and can damage DNA, proteins, and cellular membranes. Antioxidants are free radical scavengers that bind to the free radical to ensure it is no longer a reactive molecule. Antioxidants are found naturally in the body in the form of enzymes but can also be consumed in a wide variety of foods, especially vegetables and fruit. The major role in antioxidant defence is fulfilled by the body's own antioxidant enzymes, specifically eNOS, MnSOD, CAT, GPX1.

Endothelial NOS (eNOS) gene: Nitric oxide (NO) is a vital molecule produced in the body that has many important roles, including helping to lower blood pressure, improve blood flow, and boost exercise performance. eNOS encodes the endothelium-derived nitric oxide synthase enzyme, which catalyses (or uncouples) nitric oxide and plays a key role in the regulation of vascular tone.

A SNP in eNOS, could affect the production of nitric oxide, which may relate to various health conditions such as migraines, hypertension, and osteoporosis. A SNP reduces nitric oxide bioavailability in the blood vessel wall. As a result, it is associated with heart and circulation issues, kidney disease and preeclampsia, which is a horrible blood pressure condition that some pregnant women get that.

An increased intake of omega fatty acids and dietary antioxidant sources can help support this SNP, as well as increased intake of foods such as spinach and other leafy greens that can help decrease the breakdown and extend the life of nitric oxide in the body. Pomegranate and beetroot, that contain nitrates and are converted naturally in the body to nitric oxide are delicious and have loads of evidence to show that they can help.

In addition to these foods, vegetables high in nitrates and antioxidants, such as carrots, celery, and broccoli, can also help increase nitric oxide levels. Garlic is another potent food that can help improve the body's manufacturing process for nitric oxide, helping the body more effectively use the nitrates it has. Food that is high in vitamin C, such as oranges, kiwi and bell peppers, can also help increase nitric oxide production. It is important to note that while nitric oxide supplements are available, it is generally recommended to get the nitric oxide you need by eating the building blocks as part of your normal diet and of course, avoid all forms of smoke and engage in regular, moderate intensity physical activity.

Manganese Superoxide Dismutase (MnSOD or SOD2) gene - This enzyme destroys the free radicals which are normally produced within cells, and which are damaging to biological systems. The enzyme thus has important antioxidant activity within the cell, especially within the mitochondria. Resveratrol, manganese and the herb echinacea have all been shown to improve the expression of this enzyme. Also, the compounds in colourful fruit and vegetables help, so eat plenty colourful fruit and vegetables.

It is important to note that MnSOD expression can also be affected by other factors such as exercise, stress, and ageing, so please do what you can to exercise and reduce your stress as well. Also, if you are a frequent flier who has this SNP, please up your intake of colourful vegetables before, during and after the flight.

Catalase (CAT) gene: CAT encodes the antioxidant enzyme, catalase, which is most active in the liver, kidney and red blood cells. The enzyme is responsible for the rapid conversion of hydrogen peroxide to water and oxygen, where one molecule of this enzyme can catalyse more than 1 million hydrogen peroxide molecules per second. Decreased CAT activity leads to increased concentrations of hydrogen peroxide, hence leading to increased oxidative stress. Eating a polyphenol-rich diet with a high intake of colourful fruit and vegetables can help. Polyphenols can also be found in cocoa, coffee, green tea, some nuts and seeds and some spices, including cloves, cinnamon, turmeric, and ginger. Adding these spices to your meals can increase your polyphenol intake.

Decrease your environmental exposure to pollution, pesticides, smoked foods and the nitrates used as a food preservative. Stopping smoking is also strongly encouraged.

Glutathione peroxidase 1 (GPx1) gene: GPX is the most abundant of the selenoperoxidase enzymes and is active in almost all tissues in the body. It is responsible for catalysing the conversion of hydrogen peroxide into water, as well as reducing fatty acid hydroperoxides and peroxynitrite using glutathione as a substrate, and thus helps to maintain redox balance.

Eating a polyphenol-rich diet with a high intake of colourful fruit and vegetables can help. Polyphenols can also be found in cocoa, coffee, green tea, some nuts and seeds and some spices, including cloves, cinnamon, turmeric, and ginger. Adding these spices to your meals can increase your polyphenol intake. Also, include good food sources of selenium (such as brazil nuts). Avoid toxin exposure from heavy metals and pesticides and stop smoking if you smoke!

Summary of the oxidative stress genes:

eNOS - increase your colourful fruit and vegetables

MnSOD - increase colourful fruit and vegetables and practice stress management

CAT - increase your colourful fruit and vegetables, focusing on polyphenols

GPX1- increase your colourful fruit and vegetables, focusing on polyphenols and selenium

Chapter 14: Genes That Infer a Higher Need for Certain Nutrients

Finally, it is advisable to assess the genes that affect your nutritional needs for essential nutrients like Vitamin D, Vitamin A and Vitamin C. Having SNPs in any of these genes may mean you need additional nutritional support while detoxing any stored metals, mycotoxins or pollutants. Remember that it is always best to be supervised by a qualified professional who will be able to use their training to guide you through the detox process and advise you on how to support your unique needs.

Vitamin D Receptors (VDR) genes: SNPs in the VDR genes, may indicate a higher need for Vitamin D3. These receptors are known to be down regulated (made less sensitive) by several kinds of infections, including Epstein Barr Virus (EBV), which most of the population has dormant, but can be active in someone with a body burden of toxins. The mould Aspergillus also down-regulates the VDR using the mycotoxin gliotoxin.

It's useful to keep in mind that while the impact of these pathogens on the VDR has been studied, other pathogens not yet studied may also impact the VDR. When there are fewer VDRs and/or they don't respond as well, the effect of vitamin D is diminished, even when the blood level of vitamin D is adequate. The best sources are the flesh of fatty fish and fish liver oils. Smaller amounts are found in egg yolks, cheese, and beef liver. Certain mushrooms contain some vitamin D2; in addition, some commercially sold mushrooms contain higher amounts of D2 due to intentionally being exposed to high amounts of ultraviolet light. You can also make your own by sunbathing.

If you have SNPs in the VDR genes, you may need a higher dose of Vitamin D in the form of a supplement to support your immune system. Do regular testing to ensure you are always in the optimal range.

25-hydroxylase 1 (CYP2R1) gene: The CYP2R1 gene provides instructions for making an enzyme called 25-hydroxylase. This enzyme carries out the first of two reactions to convert vitamin D to its active form, 1,25-dihydroxyvitamin D3, also known as calcitriol. If you have a SNP in this gene, I encourage the intake of vitamin D-rich foods and, where possible, ensure adequate sun (UV) exposure of at least 30 minutes daily for the production of vitamin

D. When sun exposure and dietary intake of vitamin D is insufficient and where serum levels are inadequate, supplementation of vitamin D will be required.

Vitamin A is essential for VDR function. The need for Vitamin A is additionally impacted by the gene BCO1

Beta-Carotene Oxygenase 1 (BCO1) gene The BCO1 gene is responsible for making a protein that is involved in the conversion of beta-carotene into retinoic acid (the active form of vitamin A) that can be used by the body. Vitamin A is crucial for your brain, immune system, skin, eyes, teeth, bones and for the formation of hormones. After digestion and absorption of the carotenoids from red, orange and yellow fruit and vegetables, they are converted the active form of vitamin A. If you have a SNP in either of the 2 BCO1 genes, you may need additional vitamin A from supplements or specific foods. Food sources of Vitamin A (not just beta-carotene from red, yellow and orange vegetables) include beef and fish liver, egg yolk, cheese and other dairy.

Fucosyltransferase 2 (FUT2) gene. The FUT2 gene may profoundly influence gut microbiota composition and your susceptibility to viral infections and chronic inflammatory disease. Vitamin B12 need can be affected by a SNP in FUT2. If you have a SNP in FUT2, you may need to increase your intake of vitamin B12-rich foods such as clams, egg yolks and beef. But you should also be more aware of the fact that your guts are more susceptible to having an imbalance of good and bad bugs.

In certain at-risk individuals; the elderly, pregnant women, vegetarians and vegans, those suffering from gastrointestinal diseases and malabsorption syndromes, as well as those taking medications such as metformin & proton-pump inhibitors, vitamin B12 supplementation may be required. Biochemical tests to consider for monitoring the adequacy of vitamin B12 levels include measuring the methylmalonic acid (MMA) metabolite in urine or blood, serum vitamin B12 and holotranscobalamin (holoTC). Approximately one-quarter of circulating cobalamin (vitamin B-12) binds to transcobalamin (holoTC) and is thereby available for the cells of the body. For this reason, holoTC is also referred to as active vitamin B-12. Clinical studies that compare the ability of holoTC and vitamin B-12 to identify individuals with vitamin B-12 deficiency (elevated concentration of methylmalonic acid) suggest that holoTC performs better than total vitamin B-12.

Glutathione S-transferase theta-1 (GSTT1) gene: Vitamin C need is genetically determined by the GSTT1 gene which is a detoxifying enzyme that contributes to the glutathione-ascorbic acid (vitamin C) antioxidant cycle. This gene is slightly different to the others in that it is not a SNP, but either it is there (insertion), or it isn't there (deletion). In the presence of the null or deletion genotype, it is important to focus on decreasing oxidative stress exposure from the environment, including avoiding high-pollution areas, weight management, and managing psycho-social stress. Increase dietary intake of vitamin C-rich foods such as chillies, kiwi fruit, guava, and citrus fruit. Supplementation with vitamin C may also be required in at-risk groups and those with poor dietary intake.

Finally, many people are sensitive to gluten and dairy.

No, it's not just a fad to be gluten free without a coeliac disease diagnosis, some people are genetically more sensitive! To find out if you are, you can assess HLA DQ2/DQ8, the genes that predispose people to Coeliac disease and gluten sensitivity. Coeliac disease (CD) is an autoimmune disorder, in which the small intestine is damaged in response to a severe gluten intolerance. Specific Human Leukocyte Antigen (HLA) genes represent the major genetic predisposition. The most important gene variants associated with susceptibility to coeliac disease are HLA DQ2.2, DQ2.5 and DQ8. A positive HLA test is indicative of genetic susceptibility but does not necessarily mean the disease will develop; however, in my experience, people who are positive for these genes who haven't developed Coeliac disease, still benefit from going gluten free.

Adult lactase deficiency is a common condition with a decrease in the ability of the epithelial cells in the small intestine to digest lactose, usually due to a decline in the lactase enzyme. After ingestion of milk or other dairy products, Individuals who suffer from this condition may experience abdominal cramps, bloating, distension, flatulence and diarrhoea. The gene you can assess for this is called Mini chromosome Maintenance Complex component 6, or MCM6 if you don't feel like saying all of that! If you have a SNP in the gene, you may have a lactase deficiency and should probably avoid dairy that contains lactose.

So now that we have covered the basics of genetics, detoxification and the definitions of what bad things are and how they affect your generally, let's move onto the specific's bad things, starting with heavy metals.

Summary of nutritional needs genes:

Vitamin D - The VDR & CYP2R1 - increase your food intake of Vitamin D, get some sunshine and possibly take a supplement

Vitamin A - BCO1 - increase your food intake of Vitamin A and possibly take a supplement

B12 - FUT2 - increase your intake of foods high in Vitamin B12 or possibly take a supplement.

Vitamin C - GSTT1 - increase your intake of foods rich in vitamin C or possibly take a supplement. HLA DQ2/DQ8 - go gluten free!

HLA – avoid gluten

MCM6 – avoid lactose (dairy)

Chapter 15: Heavy Metals and Why They Are Bad

I like to describe the minerals and metals on the periodic table as the members of a large and mostly functional but sometimes very dysfunctional family! They all have unique personalities. Some get along, and others really don't. At the family reunion, there is the crazy aunt dancing on the table, the silent cousin in the corner avoiding company, mom and dad just trying to keep everything together.

The ones that get along are called and support each other when it comes to absorption or action are called - *Synergistic*.

The ones who don't get along and compete for absorption or reduce their action are called - *Antagonistic*.

Understanding their personalities and their relationships to each other can really help YOU to understand how to get them into balance but also how someone will feel while they are burdened with them or detoxing them.

The other nutrients, vitamins and other co-factors which can also have synergy and antagonism, are more like family, friends or colleagues.

The good news is that when you understand the personalities of the elements, you can assess them correctly and then create balancing programs that are more effective and do no harm.

An example that may help you visualise things is the relationship between calcium and potassium and the effect this relationship has on thyroid hormone metabolism.

Calcium's nature is sedentary and hard – think about an oyster shell. Potassium is the internal cellular worker that needs a healthy cellular membrane for hormones like the thyroid hormone thyroxine to move through the membrane, where potassium can act on it. If there is too much calcium, it creates a less flexible membrane, thus making it difficult for potassium to get the thyroxine it needs to create energy. Potassium is also a sensitive mineral that is excreted during times of stress.

So, if we factor in the high calcium and the low potassium, the resulting effect would be that of a low metabolism with very similar symptoms of under active thyroid. You would balance this by addressing the underlying cause of the imbalance, the stress and adrenals while adding nutrients such as vitamins K and E and minerals like magnesium that due to their synergistic relationship with calcium, would balance it and help the body retain potassium. You see, the problem isn't that dietary intake of calcium is too high, it's the balance of the body controlling the minerals. We have plenty calcium stored within our bones. It is the imbalance of the deposition of calcium caused by chronic stress that needs to be addressed.

Giving potassium without addressing the underlying stress is like trying to fill a sink with the plug out; the body won't retain the potassium until the adrenals are no longer causing the body to excrete the potassium!

What make a metal a toxic metal? Heavy metals are naturally occurring elements that have a high atomic weight and a density at least 5 times greater than that of water. Their multiple industrial, domestic, agricultural, medical and technological applications have led to their wide distribution in the environment; raising concerns over their potential effects on human health and the environment. Their toxicity depends on several factors including the dose, route of exposure, and chemical species, as well as the age, gender, genetics, and nutritional status of exposed individuals. Because of their high degree of toxicity, arsenic, cadmium, chromium, lead, and mercury rank among the priority metals that are of public health significance. These metallic elements are considered systemic toxicants that are known to induce multiple organ damage, even at lower levels of exposure. Heavy metals are everywhere in our environment that everyone is exposed to them at some point. They are environmental pollutants and are all around us – in the air we breathe, in the water we drink, in the food we eat and in materials we touch. They cannot be avoided completely and are found in virtually everyone to some degree.

In most cases, we are well equipped with functioning enzymes that help to remove toxic heavy metals quickly via the kidneys and liver. Anything over the detoxification capability of the body is quickly sequestered (moved into storage) so that the metal is rendered less harmful than when it is in circulation.

An interesting fact about metals and the organ or tissue type they are most likely going to be sequestered is that each metal has a "favourite" tissue that the body prefers to store them in. You can find these details in the reference section. It's important to know the tissue type because that can help you understand how you will feel while mobilising these metals from storage. A quick example here is that Lead (Pb) goes into the bones and nervous tissue. When people are detoxing lead, they tend to get unexplained joint pain. The joints "flare up" as the lead moves out of the bones through the joints. The pain can be severe. It lasts about four days and then passes. Interestingly, there is often no inflammation, no redness, just pain!

Another thing to remember about metals is that not all metals are overtly bad or good. Some metals, such as copper, cobalt, iron, nickel, magnesium, molybdenum, chromium, selenium, manganese and zinc, have functional roles which are essential for various diverse physiological and biochemical activities in the body. However, even these useful metals can be harmful in high doses.

Other metals such as cadmium, mercury, lead, aluminium, mercury and arsenic have toxic effects on the body in tiny quantities, causing some acute reactions or, if the dose is low but prolonged, chronic conditions in humans.

The physician, alchemist and astrologer Paracelsus (1493–1541)—who is widely regarded as the father of toxicology—famously wrote,

> "All things are poison,
>
> and nothing is without poison,
>
> only the dose permits something not to be poisonous."

A growing body of research into the biological role of many metal ions is now proving that this insight still holds true: too much of an apparently 'good' metal is toxic. Even more surprisingly, it seems that humans and other organisms might even need some 'bad' metals to function properly. Even arsenic, the poison of choice for many murderers, is now close to qualifying as a micronutrient in animals. It seems that arsenic has a role in the metabolism of the amino acid methionine and in gene silencing. Other work suggests that it has a positive interaction with the more important micronutrient, selenium. Arsenic has also been used in the past as a medicine! It was also thought that arsenic consumption by women gave "beauty and freshness" to the skin. One of the most celebrated arsenic-based therapeutics was 'Fowler's solution', a liquid substance developed during the 1780s containing potassium arsenite. It was initially recommended as a treatment for malaria but soon gained a reputation as a general tonic, an effective treatment for eczema and other severe skin disorders, and a cure for virulent diseases such as cholera. Proving that not all bad is always bad!

Having said that... Please don't supplement Arsenic!

 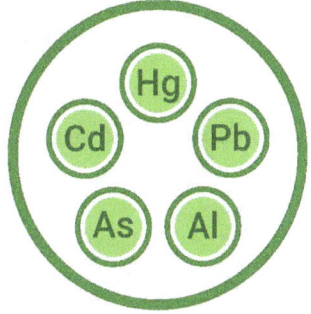

What does Heavy Metal Toxicity mean?
Toxicity is defined as being above a certain defined clinical level for some heavy metals when found using tests. This elevation is also accompanied by signs and symptoms related to the specific metal.

What does a Heavy Metal Burden mean?
A burden actually falls below a defined limit without accompanying signs and symptoms commonly associated with that specific metal. This is more common than toxicity.

Poisoning from heavy metal exposure is one thing. It's a high dose from an obvious exposure and can be immediately life-threatening. What is less obvious is toxic load and the burden it has on the body.

Each heavy metal has unique toxic effects, but in general, they do a few things to us that affect the way we function. The main mechanism of heavy metal toxicity includes the generation of free radicals to cause oxidative stress (unique to each metal), damage to biological molecules such as enzymes, proteins, lipids, and nucleic acids, neurotoxicity, as well as damage to DNA, which is key to carcinogenesis, the formation of cancer.

These bad things can significantly increase our risk of developing conditions like dementia, infertility, diabetes and cancer. They are also known to cause damage to the liver, kidneys and brain, as well as the cardiovascular, nervous and hormone systems.

In excess, and when persistent, they can affect the synthesis and actions of hormones essential for managing our general health. One gland profoundly affected by pollutants and metals is the thyroid.

Thyroid health can be undermined by nutritional deficiencies, particularly of iodine and selenium, or overexposure to bromine, arsenic, cadmium and mercury. It's important to measure thyroid markers like TSH, fT3, fT4 and TPO, as well as these elements, when assessing thyroid function.

Heavy metals can damage and alter the functioning of organs such as the brain, kidneys, lungs, liver, and blood. Heavy metal toxicity can either be acute or have chronic effects. Long-term exposure of the body to heavy metals can progressively lead to muscular, physical and neurological degenerative processes that are similar to diseases such as Parkinson's disease, multiple sclerosis, muscular dystrophy and Alzheimer's disease. Also, chronic long-term exposure to some heavy metals may cause cancer. The various health effects of some heavy metals will be highlighted in their specific chapter.

Symptoms and conditions associated with heavy metal toxicity and mineral imbalances include a wide range of acute and chronic conditions, including, but not limited to:

Cognitive decline
Mood disorders (depression)
Neurological disorders (neuropathy, headaches)
Cardiac abnormalities (arrhythmias, abnormal ECG)
Diabetes
Cancer
Reproductive issues
GI concerns (vomiting, diarrhoea)
Lung issues
Renal impairment
Skin rashes
Anaemia and other haematologic disorders

I will go into the specific details on how exactly each toxin affects us in their individual reference chapter so that if you find you have excess heavy metals from a test (hair, blood or urine), you can then go straight to that chapter at the end of the book to learn more.

Metals, Haptens and Autoimmunity

Heavy metals are also associated with the cause of autoimmune conditions thanks to their ability to form really bad things called Haptens when they bind with a protein called Albumin. Haptens are small molecules that can stimulate an immune response when attached to a large carrier such as a protein, this is called a happen adduct and is recognised by the immune system as a bad thing, so it creates anti bodies to it. Once the body has generated antibodies to a hapten adduct, the hapten-carrier adduct can now stimulate an additional immune response.

As an example, Mercury has many direct and well-recognised neurotoxic effects. However, its immune effects causing secondary neurotoxicity are less well-recognised. Mercury exposure can induce immunologic changes in the brain indicative of autoimmune dysfunction, including the production of highly specific brain autoantibodies. Mercury can combine with a larger carrier, such as a protein, creating and then acting as a hapten, and this new molecule can then elicit the production of those specific antibodies that then attack the nervous tissue.

Metallothionein:

Luckily, we have internal mechanisms for ridding the body of toxic metals, through the upregulation of enzymes called metallothionein (MTs). There are at least ten known closely related metallothionein that all have an affinity for binding metals.

They act as defences against oxidative stress and toxic metal toxicity. Zinc increases MT production and may support toxic metal clearance. MT's are a good thing!

People who would benefit from a heavy metal test:

People who smoke or are around habitual smokers

People exposed to metals either through hobbies or work

People who live in older homes where metals may be present in the paint or water pipes

Consider a test if you have low energy, chronic pain or brain fog.

If you present with health issues that could result from nutritional deficiencies or imbalances in essential elements

If you have any metal fillings/implants in your body, especially your mouth

What is a Heavy Metal Detox?

If the body is constantly detoxifying, why would there be such a thing as a "heavy metal detox?" A heavy metal detox is a lifestyle program designed to enhance how the body naturally removes toxins, specifically heavy metals.

This often includes a nutritional focus on nutrients specifically involved in the detox processes (protein, sulphur) and scavenging free radicals (antioxidants, like glutathione and vitamin C). It also typically involves following an extra clean lifestyle for a time to minimise the inflow of toxins to allow the body to focus instead on toxins that may be stored in tissues (and causing problems) from past exposures.

Often also included are lifestyle practices such as sweating through exercise and sauna and sometimes stress reduction techniques. They may also involve consuming some kind of substances that bind to toxins to either help remove them from the body or prevent their reabsorption by the intestines.

Chapter 16: Testing for Heavy Metals

Metals and minerals can be measured in various sample types, including blood, urine, hair and stool. However, there are multiple variables that impact which sample type is most appropriate, including when and how you were exposed, the dose, time span of exposure, and route of exposure. Also, remember that the body tends to remove as much as possible from circulating blood, as quickly as possible, and if there is excess that it cannot clear, it stores it for later detoxification, adding to the total body burden.

Assessment of tissue accumulation of toxic metals, or "body burden", is challenging. It is almost impossible, without doing a biopsy of the tissue that in which the metal is stored in. However; you can test to assess both current and potential past exposures. Current exposure would be seen in the blood and morning urine. Past exposure could be assessed through hair and through a challenge test, where a chelator is used to push metals out of storage for a better assessment. You can assess the body's ability to detox by assessing urine, hair, and stool.

My personal go-to tests include hair, blood, urine, and a test to assess the genetic SNP's that affect the detoxification of heavy metals discussed in the previous chapters. But remember, although I am suggesting certain tests, your practitioner may use other, equally useful tools to assess you.

Assessing through Hair Tissue Mineral Analysis (HTMA):

Hair analysis is a somewhat controversial tool, but I have found it invaluable in assessing not only heavy metals, but also the nutritional elements. Let's discuss the controversy first. I find it amazing that we can assess the dietary habits of the 5,200-year-old "Ice Man" using hair analysis or reveal the possibility of Napoleon suffering arsenic poisoning or that Michelangelo may have suffered lead poisoning, but that some still think it to be an unreliable tool for assessing living people. Hair analysis is used worldwide by many institutions, universities, and government sources. Ideally, to get more reliable results, the laboratories must be Federally, and state licensed.

Most detractors of hair analysis fail to understand numerous points about Hair Analysis or its history. These points include:

Hair analysis has a long history (over 60 years) in soil, plant, animal, and human nutrition.

Hair analysis is a "tissue biopsy" used for "cellular" nutritional/toxic elemental screening.

Hair analysis is recognised by the Environmental Protection Agency (EPA) for toxic harmful element screening.

Hair analysis is NOT a medical diagnostic test, as many continually imply.

Hair analysis is a nutritional screening tool that may infer potential manifestations based on long-standing nutrient/disease associations (i.e., low calcium may infer a potential for osteoporosis, high lead can infer exposure to that metal, etc.).

Not to be redundant, but I need to reiterate this important critical point. Hair Analysis is a nutritional screening tool that may, based on well-known nutrient/disease associations (e.g., low calcium/osteoporosis), produce INFERRED POTENTIALS (or metabolic trends) for a health condition like poor digestion or thyroid and adrenal health issues. It is NOT used to diagnose any disease; only your healthcare professional can DIAGNOSE any disease using further testing.

Most of the controversy stems from institutions, associations, or individuals who know nothing about nutrition or hair tissue mineral analysis. One of the main issues brought up is the issue of contamination of the sample. Although some obvious contamination can occur, through medicated shampoos, lead-based hair dyes, and such, I query how the hair sample can be contaminated on a person's head, without the person also being contaminated by the source? I have found that if you follow the collection protocol below, you will get reliable results!

If you are choosing to do an HTMA, please ensure you collect the sample properly to secure accurate results from the lab.

Hair analysis collection protocol:

Scalp hair is the preferred choice for a hair tissue mineral analysis. Scalp hair is one of the most metabolically active tissues of the body and, as such, provides the most accurate metabolic blueprint. If scalp hair is unavailable, pubic may be used as a last resort. Don't mix hair sources, so if you are using scalp hair, only use scalp hair!

The hair sample must be untreated hair, which includes permed or bleached. If all of the hair has been chemically treated, wait until sufficient new (virgin) growth has emerged to allow collection. This is normally four weeks for one-half inch of hair growth. If you have dyed your hair darker with modern dyes, wait for at least six washes before cutting the sample. Modern hair dyes don't seem to have an effect on minerals in the hair shaft. Henna and "natural" hair dyes and dyes containing lead, do affect the results, so please wait for new growth or submit a pubic hair sample.

Make certain your shampoo isn't medicated with Zinc or selenium, as this may affect the results. Wash your hair to remove all gels, oils, hair creams, and environmental contaminants, and allow your hair to dry thoroughly prior to collection. Damp hair will interfere with the required sample weight required for the analysis. To eliminate the potential for any other contamination, do not use any other treatments after shampooing, such as rinses and/or other treatments. Do not use any aerosol sprays such as deodorants or air fresheners prior to collecting the hair sample. Keep your environment as clean as possible!

Ensure that you utilise high high-grade stainless steel scissors or thinning shears and cut the hair as close to the scalp as possible. DO NOT damage the skin or pull the hair out by the root.

Collect from the "collection area" as indicated by the illustration. Take each sample in small portions (only 10-15 strands of hair) from at least five or more different locations of on the scalp. You can use as many locations as you want (within the collection area) to make certain the collection is not noticeable. As the hair represents "time," please only submit the inch closest to the scalp and discard the length afterward that; that information would be irrelevant and would make the results less reliable. This portion of the hair is reflective of the most recent metabolic activity for the past 90 days. If your hair is shorter than 1 ½ inches, you can use that as well. Each half-inch of hair reflects metabolic activity for approximately 30 days. For example, ½ inch = 30 days, 1 inch = 60 days and 1 ½ inch = 90 days.

The length of the collected hair should not exceed one and one-half inches (1 ½ inches). Keep the one and one-half inches closest to the scalp (root) and discard the rest. For a quick reference, the "rectangular" box where you place the sample on the weight scale is approximately 1 ½ inches. Again, do not pull your hair out by the root – cut the hair as close to the scalp as possible without damaging the skin.

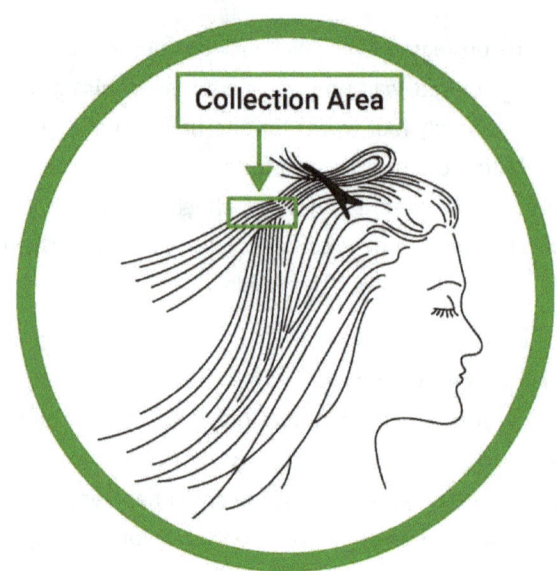

Make sure you collect enough hair. A "Hair Weight Scale" will be included with your kit to ensure a sufficient amount of hair is collected. Please use the scale! The scale is a heavy piece of paper in which you fold the sides down to provide the fulcrum point to achieve the proper weight. The weight averages approximately 125 milligrams or a tablespoon full of hair. When placing each hair sample onto the scale in the designated area, make certain the scale "tips" firmly, indicating a sufficient amount has been acquired. It is also fine acceptable to place an extra small sample onto the scale to ensure a sufficient weight is collected. An insufficient amount of hair will cause laboratory delays.

After collecting a sufficient weight of dry hair, place the hair directly from the weight scale into the hair specimen envelope (the smaller envelope) provided in your hair analysis kit. Seal the envelope with the glue flap only. Do not use plastic bags in place of the standard paper envelopes to hold the hair specimen. In addition, do not use staples, paper clips, adhesive tape, aluminium foil, or other metal and paper material of any kind to seal, secure, or wrap the hair envelope and/or the hair specimen contained within.

What I love about hair analysis is that it is non-invasive (a haircut), it is relatively cheap, and it shows an average of what the body has been exposed to or has tried to detox, over the past few months. I refer to hair analysis as looking at a ticker tape of information over time. You can see toxic exposure and assess the pattern of the elements. These patterns are controlled by and affect the nervous and hormonal systems, so that you can get an idea of general health all from a simple hair sample. From there, you can be guided to further, more directed diagnostic tests.

HTMA is limited to long-term exposure and cannot tell you about recent exposure; for that, you would need blood or urine. If a heavy metal such as arsenic was ingested, then the hair, by virtue of its normal development and growth, could not reveal the exposure until after it has been incorporated into the hair shaft. Therefore, it would take a minimum of 2-4 weeks for this to begin to occur.

During the lab assessment process, when a heavy metal is found above a certain level in a specimen being analysed, the test results for that specimen are flagged, and the entire specimen is automatically placed on hold for verification. The verification or recheck process involves the retesting of the specimen on a completely independent analytical run, which involves preparing another testing sample from the same original submittal specimen.

After the elevated level has been verified and the report has been sent to the practitioner, the next logical step is to rule out the possibility of an external source that may have inadvertently contaminated the sample before it was received in the laboratory, we do this by testing a pubic hair sample if possible. A low level in a pubic sample retest may reveal that the high level from the original scalp sample was due to the possibility of external contamination. However, if the pubic sample test is also elevated, then it would lead to the suspicion that an excess body burden does exist.

The practitioner should always take further steps when finding a markedly elevated heavy metal in a patient's HTMA results. If an external contamination has been ruled out, the next step would be to determine if the exposure is on-going or if the exposure occurred in the past. As mentioned before, HTMA is limited and cannot determine when the exposure took place, so a blood or urine test would indicate an on-going exposure. If a recent exposure is confirmed, then the source of the heavy metal should be sought and eliminated as quickly as possible.

If the blood or urine levels are not elevated, then the HTMA results would indicate an exposure from some time in the past. And since heavy metals are very quickly sequestered into tissues so, the exposure could have been from months or even years prior. It should be noted that the estimated half-life of some heavy metals in the body can be up to fifteen years. Considering this, the practitioner would then have to take a careful and thorough history to find the possible source. Unfortunately, sometimes, the source may never be identified.

The results often come with computer-generated reports. They also require some interpretation by the prescribing practitioner. When assessing the results, don't just look at the overt highs and lows, but also the relationships between the various nutrients and metals. This is where we can infer the potentials for hormonal imbalance as well as the effect of the toxins on the nutrients.

Here is a brief overview of relationships between the minerals, noting that there is a lot more information that your provider would be able to use, so this is more for guidance:

Calcium in relation to Phosphorus - when calcium is elevated in relation to phosphorus, this can infer fatigue but also poor digestion of proteins due to the stomach being less acidic than it should be. This is common due to the effects of stress and aging.

Calcium is heavy and sedentary, whereas phosphorus, explodes on contact with air. They are the opposites when it comes to energy, which is why high calcium in relation can cause fatigue in the body. The main primary food source of phosphorus is animal protein, so either the diet or digestion would need further investigation to balance these nutrients. People with a radio that is high, tend to be more prone to viral conditions.

Low calcium in relation to phosphorus may indicate low calcium overall, and this can lead to issues with the nervous system as well as bone health. People with a very low calcium-to-phosphorus ratio are also more prone to bacterial infections.

Calcium, in relation to Magnesium - is often referred to as the "Blood sugar" ratio. Calcium is required for the release of insulin from the pancreas, and Magnesium inhibits insulin secretion. Magnesium is also necessary to keep calcium in solution. Both high and low ratios indicate poor glucose metabolism and would require further investigation.

Calcium in relation to Potassium - this relationship is often referred to as the "Thyroid" relationship because calcium and potassium play a vital role in regulating thyroid activity.

High calcium in relation to potassium can indicate a sluggish thyroid. This would be seen as fatigue, brittle nails, dry skin, cold sensitivity, and weight gain. Further testing would be required. Look for overt low thyroid activity, but also pay attention to low normal ranges if the person has symptoms!

A very low Calcium to potassium could be due to calcium being low overall but also due to potassium being very high. This is an indicator of stress. In this case, address the adrenal health.

Another adrenal relationship can be seen in the relations between sodium and potassium and sodium and magnesium. These are discussed below

Sodium in relation to Potassium - The Sodium and potassium ratio is very dramatically referred to as the "Life/death" ratio as it needs to be in balance for normal average body functioning. Sodium is normally typically extracellular, while potassium is normally intracellular. If the ratio of these minerals is unbalanced, it indicates important physiological malfunctions within the cells. This ratio is related to kidney, liver, and adrenal gland function, and an imbalanced sodium/potassium ratio is associated with heart, kidney, liver, and immune deficiency diseases.

This ratio is intimately linked to adrenal gland function and the balance between aldosterone (mineralocorticoid) and cortisone (glucocorticoid) secretion. When sodium is very high on relation to potassium, this infers inflammation and adrenal imbalance or very high adrenaline. A high ratio can also be associated with angry outbursts, asthma, allergies, and kidney and liver problems. Having said this, a high sodium/potassium ratio is considered preferable to a low sodium/potassium ratio.

A moderately low ratio infers kidney and liver dysfunction, allergies, arthritis, adrenal exhaustion, digestive problems, or deficiency of hydrochloric acid. You would have to assess symptoms or need to investigate further to find out which one is relevant.

A very low ratio, less than one on the report, infers a tendency towards heart problems, arthritis, and kidney and liver disorders. Further investigation is required.

Sodium in relation to Magnesium - The sodium and magnesium ratio is also referred to as the adrenal ratio because sodium levels are directly associated with adrenal gland function. Aldosterone, a mineral corticoid adrenal hormone, regulates the retention of sodium in the body. In general, the higher the sodium level, the higher the aldosterone level.

This ratio is also a measure of energy output, because the adrenal glands are a major significant regulator (along with the thyroid gland) of the rate of metabolism. A high ratio of sodium to magnesium indicates potentially excessive activity of the adrenal cortex or very high stress levels. A very low ratio can indicate burnout.

A couple of factors which may modify the interpretation of the adrenal ratios include:

Mercury or cadmium toxicity, or an elimination of these metals which can affect the sodium/potassium ratio. Sometimes, a sodium/potassium ratio will be worse on a retest, but the patient feels better. This is because some other mineral or mineral ratio on the chart has improved, such as the elimination of cadmium or copper, or, thanks to the normalisation of another ratio, the elimination of a heavy toxic metal, the electrolytes have been lost in the process. This is usually transient and will balance over time.

Zinc in relation to Copper - I refer to these as the male-to-female relationship as the nutrients correlate to the male and female hormones.

A high zinc/copper ratio can be indicative of a zinc dominance or dominance of the male hormones, or an oestrogen deficiency, but it can also infer copper toxicity as the copper displaces zinc, making it less bio available. This can be tricky to interpret, but if you go to the reference section on copper, there is a checklist of symptoms that can help you determine if you are copper toxic or copper deficient.

Symptoms and conditions often associated with a high zinc to copper ratio may include bacterial infections, atherosclerosis, female problems, high cholesterol, and skin problems like acne but can also indicate oestrogen dominance from the hidden copper toxicity. Further testing or evaluation of the symptoms would be required.

A low zinc to copper ratio is indicative of a copper dominance and a possible copper toxicity. Symptoms and conditions often associated with a low zinc/copper ratio may include viral infections, allergies, asthma, headaches, immune deficiency, female problems such as oestrogen dominance, infections, insomnia, liver problems, skin problems (acne, eczema, hives, psoriasis, skin rashes), behaviour problems, psychological problems or emotional instability. Factors that may also impact the results include copper toxicity or the loss of zinc's bioavailability, which can artificially raise the zinc level. Cadmium and copper toxicity can elevate the zinc reading. A copper level of less than 1.0 often indicates a hidden copper toxicity.

I recommend reading the reference section on copper to get the full picture!

Iron in relation to Copper - The ratio between iron and copper can give you an idea of mitochondrial health, energy utilisation as well as blood health as both these nutrients are used to make healthy blood cells. They are also both involved in cellular respiration and electron transport.

The ratio of iron to copper, either high or low, can also lead to neurological dysfunction affecting neurotransmitters and causing lipid peroxide damage (oxidative damage) within nervous tissue.

An elevation or reduction in this ratio is associated with a decrease in the utilisation of iron into haemoglobin thus you get less efficient red blood cells.

An elevated ratio of iron to copper in the hair may indicate a potential for chronic bacterial infection. This would require further investigation.

If copper is high relative to iron, this would create a low ratio in the results and can be indicative of copper interfering with many of the functions of iron metabolism and can often contribute to iron-deficiency anaemia. Copper in excess will interfere with iron absorption and decrease the utilisation of iron by the body.

A low ratio is hence reflective of a positive trend toward copper-induced anaemia. This can lead to increased free radical production, particularly lipid peroxidation, that which can lead to oxidative stress and mitochondrial damage

A low ratio can be associated with iron deficiency as well as thyroid disturbance. We can see that even a small amount of mercury can have a profound effect of the nutrients Iron and Selenium!

Assessing metals through Full blood sample and Packed Red blood cells (RBC):

Whole or full complete blood is excellent for assessing cadmium and lead toxicity but also for evaluating recent exposure to other metals. This can be done at almost any blood lab. You can use venous blood, or you can use a lab that analyses dried blood spots from capillary blood. Capillary blood comes from a pinprick from your finger and is often considered an easier option for testing.

Packed red blood cells is a blood test where the blood is drawn from the arm and then spun so that the red blood cells can be separated from the rest of the blood. This is a great test to assess whether the exposure has started to affect biological functioning. If there are heavy metals in the red blood cells, then they are most likely also in other tissues.

This test measures blood levels of 4 common toxic metals and 8 eight nutrient elements in whole blood but also in the cell walls of the red blood cells. This profile is ideal for patients suspected of toxic metal exposure as well as common mineral imbalances. It is more invasive than a hair analysis and will need someone to draw and centrifuge (spin at high speed to separate the blood components) the sample.

The following markers are assessed in various components of the blood in alignment with the medical literature and/or National Health and Nutrition Examination Survey (NHANES) reporting.

Lead (whole blood)
Mercury (whole blood)
Arsenic (whole blood)
Cadmium (whole blood)
Chromium (whole blood)
Copper (plasma)
Magnesium (RBC)
Manganese (whole blood)
Potassium (RBC)
Selenium (whole blood)
Vanadium (whole blood)
Zinc (plasma)

Assessing metals through Urine pre and post-challenge:

Urine is an excellent, non-invasive way to assess metals. Be sure to follow the pre-testing dietary guidelines so as not to measure an accidental food exposure. The most common food advice is to avoid shellfish for the week before doing the test. The instructions will be in the kit.

Measuring urine heavy metals is an accepted method for assessing the presence of heavy metals in an individual. A random sample (without a flushing agent) done first thing in the morning, is excellent for showing current exposures because it reflects the level of heavy metals in the bloodstream during the hours immediately before bladder voiding. A sample taken after using a heavy-metal-mobilising agent (prescribed by your healthcare provider) provides a reflection of total body burden. By using both the pre- and post-flush testing, you will gain more information that cannot be acquired by other means, including identification of current exposures to lead and mercury, which is critical for proper treatment.

Conducting pre-flush testing is also currently the only means of clearly identifying cadmium toxicity. In addition, pre- and post-challenge testing allows the clinician to determine which chelating agent is the most effective for the patient; and if oral agents are employed, possible absorption problems can be identified. Since these benefits are not realised with only post-flush testing, it is recommended that clinicians test both before and after a chelation challenge.

Analysis of the levels of toxic metals in urine after the administration of a metal detoxification agent is a potentially objective way to evaluate the accumulation of toxic metals in the body tissues and hence the burden on the body as a whole. Acute metal poisoning is rare and is better evaluated through a whole blood test. More common, however, is a chronic, low-level exposure to toxic metals that can result in significant retention in the body that can be associated with a vast array of adverse health effects and chronic disease.

I won't go deeper into the various chelating agents in this book, that information would require a prescriber to administer, and they probably already know the form they need and the doses. My focus in this book will be on the synergistic and antagonistic nutrients you can use to push out the metals you have found, or that stimulate MT.

I like to use these pre and post challenge urine tests along with hair and blood to fully assess whether someone has toxicity or a burden from heavy metals and to keep track of their ability to detox effectively.

Assessing metals through Faecal (Poop) metal tests:

Faecal tests for heavy metals are available from various laboratories and can be used to evaluate the presence of toxic metals in a stool sample. These tests can reveal how many metals are moving through and out of the body

The natural route of metal detoxification is monitored for the presence of toxic metals in faeces. I use poop testing on children along with a hair test, or if I find a high level of a metal in hair, blood, or urine, I like to confirm in the stool. Also, you can use the stool to monitor detoxification.

Assessing through Dried blood and Urine

Blood spots or urine dried on filter paper strips are a convenient and practical way to test essential and toxic elements that are in the blood at the moment in time but also what is being excreted into the urine.

Dried blood requires a few spots of blood from your finger and is a convenient alternative to liquid whole blood testing for elements and is preferable to serum testing for certain elements that are found predominantly in red blood cells. Dried urine tests for elements using a simple, two-point (morning and night) urine collection, into which filter paper strips are dipped and then allowed to dry. Filter strips containing the dried urine are then shipped to the Laboratory, where the elements are extracted from the filter strips and tested for elements.

So now you have tested and found a metal! Oh NO! Don't worry; just head to the reference page and get to know your metal and how you can get it out of you!

What to do (in general) when you find metals in your body

- Remove the source where possible
- Make sure phase 3 is healthy
- Use a binder, like silica, clay or charcoal

- Support glutathione and methylation and phase 2 in general
- Up-regulate metallothionein
- Sweat

Chapter 17: Mould

Mould is everywhere!!! Mould is an ancient organism that's part of the fungi family. It grows indoors as well as outdoors. Not all moulds are bad all the time. If you think of metals as close family members and vitamins as the cousins of that family, mould is the stranger that lurks in the shadows. Not all are bad, but most, you don't want to meet alone in a dark and damp alley! I have a very healthy respect for just how deadly mould can be. I mentioned my exposure in the introduction, but I didn't give the details, except about the nosebleeds, so here they are.

I had 3 years of my life where I would house sit for someone in winter and then move to another spot for the other 6 months of summer. Within a month or so of moving into the house sit, I had an asthma attack. I didn't have asthma, so this was very strange. At around the same time, a couple I knew well, moved into the house that was diagonally across the street from me. Within a few weeks, they were both suffering from severe allergies and sinus issues. Anyway, I moved out after 6 months and the asthma I had developed resolved. YAY. Then I moved back, and the asthma came back. I want to make it clear that the house I was staying in was not damp. It didn't have the usual suspects like visible mould etc. But the house across the road, now that was covered in mould. The couple moved out and they got better, and a new couple moved in and got sick.

After the 3rd year of getting asthma like symptoms from that house sit, I never went back. I then moved into the house that gave me the nose bleeds. That house was cold and damp and had a very musty smell around the kitchen. I lived in that house, not knowing that I was being affected by the mould, for a few years. Moaning about weight gain and aches and pains and of course the nose bleeds.

One day, I had returned from travelling, and I went shopping. I hadn't been in my car for a while, and it had been out in the rain while I was away. Some of the water had leaked into the boot. I opened it to put my shopping in and thought "why can I smell cheese"? The next day, that cheesy smell was worse, so I felt around and felt the damp. But then, I put my hand into the wheel well and pulled out, what used to be a magazine, that was now damp mould food and was covered in black mould! I was touching it, breathing it and basically getting the worst exposure to all the bad compounds that mould can produce. I rushed off to my clinic and had a glutathione drip, but sadly, with the years of accumulated toxins, I was overpowered and ended up hospitalised twice from that exposure. The first time I was having little seizures, but they were bad enough that I couldn't form words. The second time I was vomiting uncontrollably as my vagus nerve was being attacked. I can't explain just how awful these experiences were, but I can tell you, mould can be deadly! I lived with almost every symptom of mould toxicity for years before I cleared myself and recovered.

Moulds affect us through exposure to spores and fragments that can stimulate an allergic response, as well as the secondary toxic metabolites they produce such as volatile compounds (that wet dog smell) which can be a serious health hazard, and mycotoxins, which by their very name... are toxic. Moulds can also grow in us, compounding the effects as they colonise us and potentially produce these toxins in us!

The main symptoms include but are not limited to:

- Allergies
- Cognitive difficulties (brain fog, poor memory, anxiety, suicidal thoughts)
- Pain (especially abdominal pain, but can include muscle pain like fibromyalgia)
- Unexplained weight gain or weight loss
- Numbness and tingling in extremities or other areas of the body
- Metallic taste in the mouth
- Vertigo or dizziness
- Tinnitus (ringing in the ears)
- Digestive issues (especially limited tolerance to food, persistent bloating, diarrhoea)
- Significant fatigue that interferes with daily activities
- Changes in mood
- Excessive thirst and dehydration, bed-wetting in children and Excessive urination
- Symptoms that resemble hormone imbalances (hair loss, rashes)
- Increased susceptibility to infections... and more

A - Toxic moulds intentionally harm other living things as a means of survival or when they feel threatened. They produce micro-toxins and other poisonous chemicals.

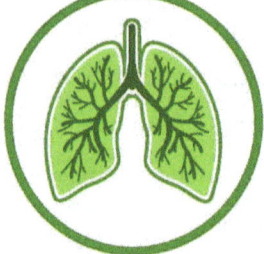 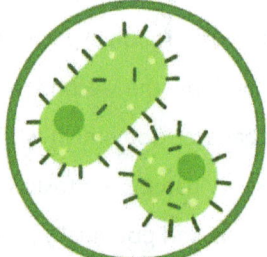

B - These moulds may affect people who have certain allergies or asthma. They possibly can cause an allergic reaction in individuals without allergies if exposed for a long period of time.

C - These opportunistic pathogens most commonly attack people with a suppressed immune system. Infants and the elderly are at the greatest risk.

They are classified as Hazard class A, B and C depending on their action on the body.

They grow in any environment that has some source of moisture. Having a relative humidity above 55% is enough moisture for mould to grow even without overt water damage. You can measure your homes humidity using a hydrometer. If your humidity goes above 55%, there are actions you can take to lower it, this is discussed a little later in the book.

We can also get exposed via certain foods, especially leftovers and fermented foods, through leaks and condensation in our homes and cars or even in the buildings we work or are schooled in! I have had a few re-exposures while travelling and staying in hotels that may not be aware of just how toxic mould is, so I am constantly having to go through the process of removing the impacts and I am sure you will also have to.

Outside, moulds are an important part of the ecosystem. They help break down plant and animal matter. When mould grows inside, it can sometimes be problematic. It can cause allergies and infections in some people. Multiple types of mould can grow in the same area.

You can't always tell the difference between types of mould without testing. Fortunately, you don't need to know the type of mould to get rid of it. Having said that, please NEVER clean mould by spraying it with bleach. This causes it to react with a flurry of mycotoxins, and people often get worse after cleaning mould. Rather, get a professional to assess and rehabilitate it for you.

Mould exposure is not an emergency for most people. This can be confusing when a whole family is exposed and only one person suffers extremely, while the others get no symptoms or only a few irritating symptoms.

Mould can affect our health in several ways. Reactive spores and fragments, mycotoxins and volatile organic compounds (VOCs), can all cause health issues, and you may have 1 or all 3 at play!

Mould affects us through:

- Disruption of the liver pathways
- Hormone disruption
- Neuro inflammation and brain shrinking
- Autonomic dysfunction
- Mast cell activation
- Malabsorption/nutrient deficiencies
- Dysbiosis/sick microbiome
- DNA damage
- Chronic immune activation
- Cell danger response
- Mitochondrial induced apoptosis (cell death).
- To name just a few!

Mould can trigger Chronic Inflammatory Response Syndrome - CIRS:

Chronic Inflammatory Response Syndrome (CIRS) is a progressive, multi-system, multi-symptom illness characterised by exposure to biotoxins. The ongoing inflammation can affect virtually any organ system of the body and if left untreated becomes debilitating.

Patients with CIRS are often misdiagnosed as having depression, anxiety, post-traumatic stress disorder, and somatisation. Somatisation is the expression of psychological or emotional factors as physical (somatic) symptoms. For example, stress can cause some people to develop headaches, chest pain, back pain, nausea or fatigue.

Other symptoms can mimic Alzheimer's, Parkinsonism, allergy, fibromyalgia, and chronic fatigue syndrome, among others. Treating patients for these seemingly diverse conditions do not improve their symptoms of CIRS, although effective therapies for CIRS exist.

Treatment would require you to identify the exposure and treat that first, then work with the microbiome and mitochondria, then supporting detoxification if needed. Ideally this would be done under the care of someone with experience!

To accurately diagnose CIRS, the ideal test would be NeuroQuant Analysis. NeuroQuant® software processes data from an MRI brain scan to calculate accurate measurements of the brain structure volumes and compare to established norms based on age, sex and cranial volume. These measurements can determine which parts of your brain are atrophied or shrunk, are asymmetrical, or even deformed. Given that cognitive symptoms are found in 94% of CIRS patients, to date the NeuroQuant Analysis remains the best measure of objective central nervous system injury from CIRS. The automated Analysis reads your brain's volume and grey matter metrics to analyse for "mould" points, Lyme points, and other conditions. It can be used in diagnosis as well as assessing response to treatment.

Spores and Fragments:

The spores and mould fragments can irritate some people's immune systems; this generally results in itching of the eyes, nose, ears, throat, and skin. Coughing and asthma are also common. In severe cases, mould can trigger Mast cell activation syndrome or MCAS. MCAS is a condition in which the patient experiences repeated episodes of the symptoms of anaphylaxis, allergic symptoms such as hives, swelling, low blood pressure, difficulty breathing and severe diarrhoea.

Other common symptoms are:
- Runny nose and congestion
- Eye irritation

- Sneezing
- Coughing
- Sore throat
- Skin rash
- Headache
- Lung irritation
- Wheezing

Tests for moulds and the reactions to moulds and spores:

Get a professional to inspect your home and environment. The gold standard testing is called the Environmental Relative Mouldiness Index (ERMI) which is a research tool developed by EPA scientists for estimating mould contamination. The results of the index can be used to estimate the amount of mould and some of the types of mould present.

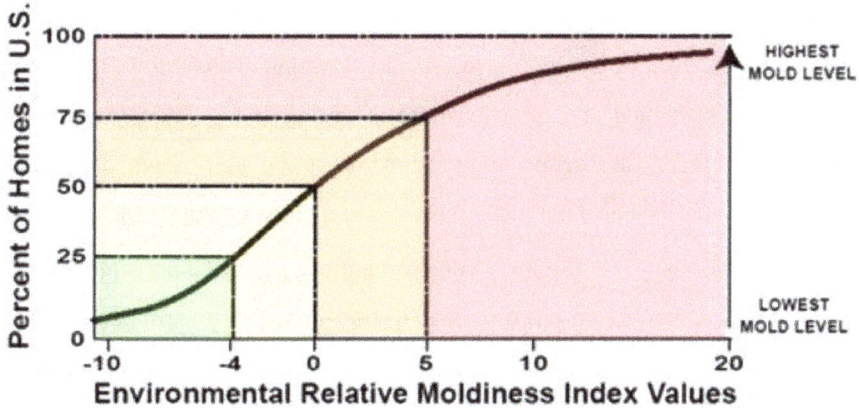

The ERMI score is the difference between Group 1 (bad) and Group 2 (good) moulds. ERMI scores range between -10 (really good) and +20 (really bad.)

There is no hard and firm line on where good ends and bad begins although scores above 8 are generally considered unhealthy.

An ERMI score is sometimes not too meaningful, particularly for sensitive and high-risk people. Most people with Chronic Inflammatory Response Syndrome (CIRS) cannot tolerate an ERMI score above +2 without becoming ill. However, there are many individuals who have been very ill and are extremely sensitive. They often need an ERMI score as low as -1 to continue recovery. If mould is affecting your health, then you need to listen to your body because a "safe" ERMI score for the general population may not be safe for you.

For your symptoms, I would recommend testing the immune system response to the mould species. This is a blood test that looks at the immune system reactions by looking at immunoglobulins, IGE, IGG, and IGA. These are different types of immunoglobulins or antibodies produced by the immune system.

IgA (Immunoglobulin A) is primarily found in the linings of the respiratory tract, digestive system, and other mucous membranes, as well as in saliva, tears, and breast milk. It plays a crucial role in defending against infections on these surfaces and provides localised immunity. If the test is positive for IGA, it means the mould is a recent or current exposure, and the environment needs to be fixed as soon as possible.

IgE (Immunoglobulin E) IgE is associated with allergic reactions and is involved in the body's response to allergens, including mould. When the immune system identifies an allergen, it triggers the production of IgE antibodies, which bind to white blood cells called basophils, as well as mast cells, which release the itch-causing histamine. This binding leads to the release of histamine and other chemicals, causing allergic symptoms. It is quite difficult to remediate an IGE reaction, so unfortunately, if you are positive to moulds as an IGE response, then you will probably have reactions every time you get close to that mould.

IgG (Immunoglobulin G) is the most common antibody in the bloodstream and other body fluids. It plays a crucial role in providing long-term immunity against bacterial and viral infections but also to mould. IgG antibodies can cross the placenta, providing passive immunity to the foetus during pregnancy. A positive result shows past exposure to the mould and a possible reactivity to the mould.

These different types of immunoglobulins have distinct functions and are involved in various aspects of the immune response. IgA is important for mucosal immunity, IgE is associated with allergic reactions, and IgG provides long-term immunity. Testing the levels of these immunoglobulins can help diagnose certain immune disorders or allergies related to mould.

It's important to note that the interpretation of these tests should be done by healthcare professionals, as results may vary depending on individual circumstances and medical history.

A note on other possible testing options:

Other testing options are offered under various protocols. In practice, I have found that testing the environment, immune response and for mycotoxins is enough for most people and I rarely use the tests listed below as they add additional costs to the program and offer very little value with respect to how I would change treating the person using the following:

- Assess and treat the environment first
- Assess and work with the microbiome and mitochondria
- Protect against oxidative stress. Consider using Astaxanthin
- Use binders specific to the mycotoxins found
- Support bile flow and detoxification, consider a choline supplement
- Sweat (sauna)

But if a case is extremely stubborn and you have tried everything already mentioned, but they have proved less effective than usual, then the following can be considered:

Vasoactive Intestinal Polypeptide (VIP) - Normal Range: 23-63 pg/mL

Vasoactive intestinal polypeptide (VIP) is a neuro regulatory hormone with receptors in the hypothalamus of the brain. Low VIP levels are present in mould illness patients. This leads to unusual shortness of breath, especially in exercise. With respect to the digestive system, VIP seems to induce smooth muscle relaxation (lower oesophageal sphincter, stomach, gallbladder), stimulate secretion of water into pancreatic juice and bile, and cause inhibition of gastric acid secretion and absorption from the intestinal lumen, which can lead to chronic, watery diarrhoea.

VIP replacement therapy, when used according to a strictly administered protocol by a registered healthcare provider, has proven to be effective in returning some chronically fatigued patients back to a normal life. Do not use VIP if you are exposed to mould (with ERMI values greater than 2), if you fail a VCS test or if you have a MARCoNS present in your nose. MARCoNS (Multiple Antibiotic Resistant Coagulase Negative Staphylococci) is an antibiotic resistant staph infection that resides deep in the nose. MARCoNS are very slow growing however, can have such an effect on health leading to chronic fatigue, hormonal imbalances, and more.

MSH - Melanocyte Stimulating Hormone - Normal Range: 35-81 pg/mL

In mould illness, MSH will be too low in over 95% of patients. This may mean increased susceptibility to mould illness, ongoing fatigue, pain, hormone abnormalities, mood swings, and much more.

TGF Beta-1 - Transforming Growth Factor Beta-1 - Normal Range: <2380 pg/ml

This protein helps control the growth and division (proliferation) of cells, the process by which cells mature to carry out specific functions (differentiation), cell movement (motility), and the self-destruction of cells (apoptosis). The TGF Beta-1 protein is found throughout the body and plays a role in development before birth, the formation of blood vessels, the regulation of muscle tissue and body fat development, wound healing, and immune system function (especially regulatory T-cells).

C4a - Normal Range: 0-2830 ng/ml

C4a has become the inflammatory marker of greatest significance looking at innate immune responses in those with exposure to Water Damaged Buildings (WDB). An initial rise of plasma levels is seen within 12 hours of exposure to biotoxins, and sustained elevation is seen until definitive therapy is initiated.

HLA DR - Your Genes

Human Leukocyte Antigens (HLAs) are found on the surface of nearly every cell in the human body. They help the immune system tell the difference between body tissue and foreign substances. Almost a quarter of the normal population is genetically susceptible to chronic mould illness.

Antigliadin (AGA) IgA/IgG - Normal Range: 0-19

Antigliadin (AGA) antibodies are produced in response to gliadin, a small protein that is part of gluten, biologically active of wheat, barley and rye. These antibodies were thought at one time to be specific for Celiac Disease. Antigliadin antibodies are found in over 58% of children with biotoxin-associated illness.

ACTH/Cortisol - Normal Range: ACTH - 8-37 pg/mL; Cortisol - a.m. 4.3-22.4 / p.m. 3.1-16.7 ug/dL

ACTH is a hormone released from the anterior pituitary gland in the brain. Cortisol is a steroid hormone produced by the adrenal cortex, which is the outer part of the adrenal gland. The adrenal glands are located on top of both kidneys.

Early in the illness, as MSH begins to fall, high ACTH is associated with few symptoms; a marked increase in symptoms is associated with a fall in ACTH. Finding simultaneous high cortisol and high ACTH may prompt consideration of screening tumours, but the reality is that the dysregulation usually corrects with therapy.

Vascular endothelial growth factor VEGF - Normal Range: 31-86 pg/mL

Vascular endothelial growth factor (VEGF) is a substance made by cells that stimulates new blood vessel formation and increases blood flow in the capillary beds. Deficiency of VEGF is quite common and is a serious problem in biotoxin illness patients that must be corrected. If you don't have blood flow, cells begin to starve and don't work properly.

Anticardiolipins (ACLA) IgA/IgG/IgM - Normal Range: IgA - 0-12; IgG 0-10; IgM 0-9

Anticardiolipins (ACLA) are autoantibodies. IgA, IgM, and IgG are autoantibodies often identified in collagen vascular diseases such a lupus and scleroderma and are often called anti-phospholipids. An increased risk of miscarriage in the first trimester of pregnancy is commonly seen in women with the presence of these autoantibodies. They are also found in over 33% of children with biotoxin-associated illnesses.

ADH/Osmolality - Normal Range: ADH - 1.0-13.3 pg/ml; Osmolality - 280-300 mmol

Antidiuretic hormone (ADH), or vasopressin, is a substance produced naturally by the hypothalamus and released by the pituitary gland. The hormone controls the amount of water your body removes. Symptoms associated with dysregulation of ADH include dehydration, frequent urination, with urine showing low specific gravity; excessive thirst and sensitivity to static electrical shocks; as well as oedema and rapid weight gain due to fluid retention during initial correction of ADH deficits.

Matrix metallopeptidase 9 (MMP-9) - Normal Range: 85-332 ng/mL

Matrix metallopeptidase 9 (MMP-9) is an enzyme that is involved in the breakdown of extracellular matrix in normal physiological processes, such as embryonic development, reproduction, and tissue remodelling, as well as in disease processes.

Leptin - Normal Range: Male: 0.5-13.8 ng/mL; Female: 1.1-27.5 ng/mL

Leptin turns on how tightly the body holds onto fatty acids. When Leptin is high, one holds onto fatty acids and stores them in fat. This leads to rapid weight gain, and because of the high Leptin, standard approaches to weight loss like eating less and exercising more will fail. The inflammatory responses that cause Leptin levels to rise lead to patients who are chronically tired, in chronic pain, and forever overweight.

As mentioned, I very infrequently use these tests as a good history, assessment of the environment and treating the basics tends to be all you need to do. Get the bad stuff out and put the good stuff in and your body will heal itself!

Not often mentioned are the white blood cells Eosinophils and Neutrophils, which can sometimes be found out of range in random blood tests! Eosinophils will go up when there are allergic reactions that may be due to mould or parasites and neutrophils are often low in chronic mould conditions, so if you see either of these 2 out of range in a blood test, and you have symptoms, please do further testing for mould starting with the immune and mycotoxin assessments.

Chapter 18: Managing Moisture to Prevent Mould Growth

The primary reason for visible mould growth is due to condensation. The property needs ventilation and dehumidification to keep mould at bay. Simply opening the windows more often will usually reduce the risk of condensation occurring. Here are the key points to follow in order to create a healthier indoor environment.

Opening Windows in Bursts During Winter: -

Fully open the windows in ten-minute bursts during winter (front and back of the property) to create cross-ventilation. Windows should be opened more often during other seasons of the year.

Correctly Heating the Property and Humidity and Temperature Levels: -

Use a hydrometer to monitor the humidity levels in the property and keep it 55% and under during the winter - and during cold spring and autumn weather. The property should be correctly heated (18-21 Celsius or 64-70 Fahrenheit), which is critical for moisture management. Bedrooms can be 18-19 degrees Celsius, whereas living areas should be 20-21 degrees Celsius. To achieve these humidity levels, you will need to use a good quality dehumidifier of around 20-25 litres capacity.

Ways to Reduce Condensation Build-up on Window Areas During Winter Nights: -

Open the windows in the bedroom (short burst) before going to bed, and this will lower the air temperature in the room, and thereby reduce the possibility of moisture condensing on the windows during the night. Consider leaving the bedroom windows in a locked-open position during the night (even in winter), to enable a small input of air. Alternatively, (if you have them) ensure window trickle vents are permanently open. Sleeping with the bedroom door open will enable moisture from breath to escape. These types of actions will help reduce condensation forming in the bedroom during the night. If there is moisture on the windows and on the abutting walls in the morning, this should be dried using absorbent cloths. The use of a window cleaning blade and a moisture vacuum will help to dry these areas when there is excessive moisture present. You could also invest in a good dehumidifier.

Drying Washing:

Avoid Drying on Radiators and Using Heated Rails. Where possible, dry washing outdoors or use a tumble dryer. Tumble dryers must be correctly vented to the outside (not into the garage); otherwise, a condensing dryer should be used. These are the best options. Alternatively, dry washing in the sunniest room with the windows open.

As an alternative to a tumble dryer, dehumidifiers are much cheaper to run, and a good quality one will dry washing within about half a day. I would typically recommend one with a 20-25 litre capacity. Its effectiveness to dry washing will, in part, depend on the litre capacity/performance of the dehumidifier in relation to the size of the room it's operating in. Place the washing in a sunny room (ideally a smaller sized room and not a bedroom) with the windows and doors closed.

Bear in mind that for those with asthma - or who have immune-suppressed conditions - there is research that shows that there are possible risks to exacerbating such conditions when drying in-doors. As well as drying washing more quickly, from a health perspective, opening windows or running a dehumidifier is important. Certainly, do avoid drying clothes on radiators and on heated rails. Even if washing is dried on a heated rail with a cover over it, the cover won't adequately contain the moisture and it will become mouldy.

Placement of Furniture: -

Move furniture and other items away from walls, to enable airflow to all areas. Where possible, arrange furniture by the warmer internal walls, with a good-size gap between the furniture and the wall itself. Lack of airflow will cause the air behind furniture to become static, and then it is likely to 'sweat.' This in turn will cause condensation to form on the back of furniture and on the abutting wall, creating conditions for mould growth.

Decluttering and Keeping the Property Dust-Free: -

It's important to keep the property tidy and uncluttered. This will enable better airflow throughout. It's essential to keep skirting boards and other areas dust-free (including the back of furniture). This is particularly important in rooms where there has been a mould issue.

Bathroom Extraction Fans and Opening of Bathroom Windows: -

Be sure to run the bathroom extractor fan whilst showering or bathing, and for up to an hour following. The bathroom windows must be opened wide and be left open during a bath or shower, with the bathroom door closed. Leave the windows open for around 30-45 minutes (longer if you only have a small, awning style-window). Do this all year round, even in winter. It may be uncomfortable bathing in the winter with the window open, in which case they should be fully opened when finished, even on a cold winter day. The outside air will dry the tiles, walls and ceiling, and thereby help avoid mould-growth conditions. A glass cleaning wiper blade can also be used to remove excessive moisture from bathrooms tiles and shower screens.

Bathroom Sealant: -

Wetness that is left to sit on bathroom sealant will attract mould spores, and overtime mould will become embedded in it. Once black mould has attached itself to sealant, it will have to be cut away and reapplied. It is therefore important that sealant is dried with an absorbent cloth, if it doesn't naturally dry by opening the windows.

Don't dry Towels on Heated Bathroom Rails: -

Don't hang wet or damp towels on bathroom radiators or towel rails. Hanging wet towels will generate moisture that will condense on the walls and ceiling. Hanging dry towels on radiators or heated towel rails will block some of the heat that is needed for the bathroom, so if you can avoid this.

Kitchens: -

Be sure to turn on the kitchen extraction fan when cooking begins. The fan should be left on for up to an hour after the cooking has finished. If possible, close the kitchen door so that moisture doesn't escape to other areas of the property. If you have windows, they can be opened to provide additional ventilation. The opening of kitchen windows is necessary if your extraction fan is sub optimal. To limit moisture in the kitchen, cover pans with lids when cooking.

Avoid storing items above kitchen wall units, as this will block airflow to this area, which in turn will cause air to become static. For these reasons, areas such as this are more susceptible to condensation and mould growth.

Wardrobes and cupboards: -

Try to leave wardrobe doors open for at least a few hours each day, and during the time the bedroom windows are open. This will enable airflow into wardrobes. Additionally, wardrobe doors may need air-vents in them. Avoid over-packing wardrobes.

If you do get mould, remember that you can use ozone (but be careful, read up on this first because it can also be toxic) or you can get professionals who can remediate the damp.

Chapter 19: Mycotoxins

Mycotoxins are tiny toxic chemical substances that certain types of moulds produce. There are over 400 mycotoxins, most of which are cytotoxic (toxic to living cells). 11 are commonly tested for in urine and are discussed in the reference section. Mycotoxins are as small as 0.1 microns. For reference, mould spores are between 1 and 20 microns, still tiny but not as tiny as mycotoxins. This means they are invisible and can move through porous walls and ceilings!

Mycotoxins-producing moulds typically grow on either the floor or walls in a humid and confined environment or on certain foods. Unless they have colonised you, then they are made inside you!

Although they are also secondary metabolites of moulds, mycotoxins are different from the musty smell of volatile gasses that are discussed in chapter 21; they are toxins produced by the mould for 1 of 2 reasons:

1 - To protect itself from death, which is why they are released when you try to clean mould off surfaces

2 - To break things down to eat them, including you; yes, you are food!

Mycotoxins are thought to play a role in helping to prepare the substrate on which the moulds exist for digestion. They have also been found to act as defence mechanisms. This is why people who clean mould without protective gear tends to have more of an exposure Mycotoxins may be produced when the organisms are under stress, which could be related to competition/defence, or simply due to inhospitable environmental conditions.

The traditional definition of mycotoxins is that they are secondary metabolites produced by microscopic fungi that can cause disease and death in humans and other animals at low concentrations. They are so toxic that they are used in biological warfare because the fact is, although many people are sensitive to mould, spores, and off gasses, EVERYONE is affected by mycotoxins!

Like all toxicoses, the symptoms of the diseases caused by mycotoxins ("mycotoxicosis") depend on the type and amount of mycotoxin, the length of the exposure, the age and the sex of the exposed person, and many other parameters involving genetics, current health status and interactions with other physiological factors. The severity of a mycotoxicosis can be increased by stresses like starvation and alcoholism. In turn, mycotoxicosis can heighten vulnerability to microbial diseases and worsen the effects of malnutrition.

The major mycotoxins associated with human and veterinary diseases (yes, they affect your pets, too) include aflatoxin, citrinum, ergot alkaloids, fumonisins, ochratoxin A, patulin, and trichothecenes. Mycotoxins exert their toxicities with different mechanisms. For example, aflatoxins damage DNA, fumonisin is an inhibitor of cell membrane biosynthesis, and trichothecenes interfere with protein synthesis.

Mycotoxin testing is an imperfect science, but something is always better than nothing. By knowing which toxins, we or our clients and patients are exposed to and how those toxins are cleared from the body allows us to precisely target our intervention.

It is worth noting that many mycotoxins need to be cleared through multiple pathways, and detoxification is not as linear as the liver detox model — phase 1, phase 2, and phase 3 (elimination). The more targeted and precise the intervention, the better the odds that people will get better. The main route of detoxification of most mycotoxins is Glucuronidation, followed by Glutathione conjugation and Methylation; however, all 6 pathways of Phase 2 detoxification should be supported through eating the right foods or taking the right supplements.

The symptoms of mycotoxicosis can vary depending on the type of mycotoxin, the amount and duration of exposure, and individual susceptibility. Here are some common symptoms associated with mycotoxicosis:

Respiratory Symptoms: Mycotoxin exposure can lead to respiratory issues such as coughing, wheezing, shortness of breath, chest tightness, sore throat, and sinus congestion. These symptoms may resemble those of allergies or respiratory infections. Asthma-like symptoms are common.

Gastrointestinal Symptoms: Mycotoxins can cause gastrointestinal problems such as abdominal pain, diarrhoea, nausea, vomiting, and loss of appetite. These symptoms can be like food poisoning or other gastrointestinal illnesses. Weight gain or loss without changes in diet are also common. Mycotoxins can also kill off the good gut bugs so you may need to check your gut as well.

Urological symptoms: Increase in the frequency of urination is a common symptom as mycotoxins block the hormone Antidiuretic hormone, which stops us from losing too much water. If this hormone is blocked, every glass of liquid you drink will quite likely flow straight through you!

Neurological Symptoms: Some mycotoxins have neurotoxic effects and can affect the central nervous system. Neurological symptoms may include headache, dizziness, fatigue, difficulty concentrating, memory problems, mood changes (including anxiousness and depression), and sensory disturbances. There is very often a nerve pain described as "ice pick" sensations as well as tingling in the limbs. Insomnia is also very common as mycotoxins interfere with the manufacture and use of Melatonin.

Skin and Eye Irritation: Direct contact with mycotoxins or mould spores can cause skin irritation, such as redness, itching, or a rash. Exposure to mycotoxins may also lead to eye irritation, such as red, itchy, or watery eyes.

Immune System Effects: Mycotoxins can suppress the immune system, leading to an increased susceptibility to infections and other illnesses. This may result in recurrent respiratory or other infections. This is why there are often flare-ups of the bacteria Lyme and the Epstein-Barre virus.

Nose bleeds and other bleeding disorders are also common. Mycotoxins have the potential to disrupt various physiological processes in the body, including blood clotting and platelet function. As a result, exposure to certain mycotoxins can lead to bleeding disorders. Here are a few more ways mycotoxins can contribute to bleeding issues:

Inhibition of Coagulation Factors: Some mycotoxins, such as aflatoxins and ochratoxins, can interfere with the activity of coagulation factors, which are proteins involved in blood clotting. These mycotoxins may inhibit the production or function of specific coagulation factors, impairing the normal clotting process and increasing the risk of bleeding.

Platelet Dysfunction: Mycotoxins can affect platelet function, leading to platelet dysfunction. Platelets are blood cells responsible for forming blood clots. Mycotoxin-induced platelet dysfunction can result in decreased platelet aggregation, reduced clot formation, and an increased risk of bleeding.

Vascular Effects: Certain mycotoxins, like T-2 toxin and fumonisins, can cause damage to blood vessels, disrupting their integrity and function. This vascular damage can lead to increased permeability, fragile blood vessels, and a propensity for bleeding.

Disruption of Blood Coagulation Pathways: Mycotoxins may interfere with various components of the blood coagulation pathways, disrupting the delicate balance between clotting and bleeding. They can impact the activation and regulation of clotting factors, leading to an imbalance that favours bleeding.

It's important to note that the specific mycotoxin, dosage, duration of exposure, and individual susceptibility all play a role in determining the severity and type of bleeding disorder that may occur. The likelihood and extent of bleeding disorders resulting from mycotoxin exposure can vary widely.

Severe cases are typically associated with high levels of mycotoxin exposure or exposure to particularly potent mycotoxins. Many people may experience mild symptoms or no symptoms at all, even with exposure to mould and mycotoxins. If you suspect mycotoxicosis or have concerns about mould exposure, it is recommended to seek medical attention for proper evaluation and guidance.

How to test whether you have been affected by Mycotoxins:

There are a few ways to test, so let's have a look at each of them.

Visual acuity test:

Mycotoxins can affect your visual acuity. A visual acuity test is an eye exam that checks how well you see the details of a letter or symbol from a specific distance. Visual acuity refers to your ability to discern the shapes and details of the things you see. There are several different types of visual acuity tests, most of which are very simple. Depending on the type of test and where it's conducted, the exam can be performed by:

- An optometrist
- An ophthalmologist
- An optician
- A nurse
- You can also find them online

No risks are associated with visual acuity tests, and you don't need any special preparation. It is important to note, though, that other factors can also affect your visual acuity, so this is not a fully diagnostic test but can be a useful tool.

Mycotoxins urine tests:

These tests measure free (unconjugated) Mycotoxins in the urine; this is a good way to assess what your body has processed over the past few days. If you are going to do a mycotoxin test, I don't advise using glutathione for the week before the test. However, the day before the test, I do advise the following:

- Stimulate lymph drainage - you can do this by dry skin brushing, rebounding on a trampoline or getting a lymph drainage massage.
- Sauna if you have access to one. If not, then have a hot bath with a handful of Epsom salts and some lovely aroma oils.
- Then drink as little as possible without getting too uncomfortable.
- Go to bed and do the test using the first-morning urine sample.

There are now also mycotoxin antibody tests available in some countries as well; however, I have no personal experience with them yet.

Treating mould in the environment (addressing Phases 0):

Remember to always treat your exposure first:

- Reduce exposure to susceptible food and damp environments
- Get a professional to assess and treat your environment if needed
- Get a good air purifier and dehumidifier
- Always wear PPE (gloves and a mask) when cleaning any visible mould, but ideally, get someone else to clean it for you
- Get a probiotic cleaning solution; there are a few commercially available.

You can also make your own natural All-Purpose Cleaning Formula that can kill mould spores and neutralise some mycotoxins on hard surfaces with this natural formula - the recipe is in the recipe eBook on the website. This can be used as a replacement for commercial cleaning products that contain harsh chemicals and may not address all moulds.

Note that this won't remediate porous surfaces; for porous surfaces, I recommend getting professional fogging done.

Treating mould in you (addressing Phase 2):

- Assess and treat the environment first
- Assess and work with the microbiome and mitochondria
- Protect against oxidative stress. Consider using Astaxanthin
- Use binders specific to the mycotoxins found
- Support bile flow and detoxification, consider a choline supplement
- Sweat (sauna)
- Give yourself time to heal

What does detoxing mycotoxins feel like

To put it plainly, when I started detoxing mycotoxins, I felt awful! My first sauna was quite short and really kicked a load of stored mycotoxins out. It triggered inflammation and I felt sore, tired and very unwell. But I pushed through and after a few days the symptoms resolved. This happened to a lesser degree over time and now I don't experience any symptoms. But prepare yourself. If you have had a long or large exposure, you won't feel well while removing them! You will feel well eventually though, so hang in there through the bad times. Make sure you are using your binders and putting all the good stuff in so your body can heal.

Chapter 20: Volatile Organic Compounds

As mentioned, Mycotoxins are secondary metabolites, which are toxic; but there are also the Volatile organic compounds (VOCs). These produce that "wet dog" smell most people associate with damp and mould but what most people don't know, is that they are also toxic in their own way.

VOCs are substances that vaporise easily under normal room temperature conditions and have two or more actions or functions. All fungi emit blends of VOCs; the composition of these volatile blends varies with the species of fungus and the environmental situation in which the fungus is grown.

These fungal VOCs are produced as mixtures of nasty chemicals, including alcohols, aldehydes, acids, ethers, esters, ketones, terpenes, thiols, and their derivatives. These are responsible for the characteristic mouldy odours associated with damp indoor spaces. There is increasing experimental evidence that some of these VOCs have toxic properties and have been termed "volatoxins" in some research articles.

Several published studies have shown that exposure to several volatile organic compounds such as benzene and formaldehyde leads to adverse health effects, especially blood-related toxicities and the worsening of allergy/asthma. Short-term inhalation exposure to VOCs has been associated with respiratory tract irritation, headaches, and visual impairment. Inhalation and skin exposure to these compounds provide rapid entry into the body's systemic circulation, resulting in subsequent toxic effects distant from the entry route that can include damage to the liver, kidneys, and central nervous system.

Exposure to volatile organic compounds (VOC) from moulds can cause a range of symptoms, which can vary depending on the individual and the extent of exposure. Some of the main symptoms associated with VOC mould exposure include:

Respiratory Issues: Common respiratory symptoms include coughing, wheezing, shortness of breath, chest tightness, and sinus congestion. These symptoms can be particularly problematic for individuals with pre-existing respiratory conditions such as asthma or allergies.

Allergic Reactions: Mould exposure can trigger allergic reactions in some individuals. Symptoms may include sneezing, runny or stuffy nose, itchy or watery eyes, sore throat, and skin rash or hives.

Headache and Fatigue: Exposure to VOC moulds may lead to persistent headaches and general fatigue. These symptoms can impact daily functioning and overall well-being.

Irritation of the Eyes, Nose, and Throat: Moulds produce airborne irritants that can irritate the mucous membranes of the eyes, nose, and throat. This can result in red, itchy, or watery eyes, nasal congestion or runny nose, and throat irritation.

Skin Irritation: Direct contact with mould or mould-contaminated materials can cause skin irritation, such as redness, itching, or a rash. This can occur particularly if an individual has a sensitivity or allergy to the specific mould species.

Neurological Symptoms: Some individuals may experience neurological symptoms after mould exposure, although these symptoms are less common. Examples include difficulty concentrating, memory problems, dizziness, and changes in mood or behaviour.

It's important to note that the severity and duration of symptoms can vary widely among individuals. If you suspect mould exposure or are experiencing persistent symptoms, it is recommended to consult with a healthcare professional for proper evaluation and guidance. Additionally, addressing the underlying mould issue and ensuring proper remediation is crucial for reducing exposure and potential health effects.

Chapter 21: Plastics and Persistent Organic Pollutants

Is your new, fireproof furniture, or the Teflon coated pan set you bought because they made life easier, making you sick? Do you use fabric softener, scented candles and air fresheners? Well, sadly, they may be contributing to your toxic burden!

Carbon is main element that we are made from. We are carbon-based life forms. Carbon strands make organic structures. When 8 Carbon (C8) atoms linked together, this makes an incredibly strong structure, that is very hard to break down. Something we have learned over time is that household hacks and inventions that seemed ideal and useful at the time they were discovered, all become disappointingly "toxic" the more we get to know them. When plastic was first invented, we all wanted the full Tupperware set; everything was better in plastic. Now we know better! Then there was Teflon, made of 8 carbon atoms! YAY, nothing sticks to the pan! And now we know better! C8 is a persistent organic pollutant that can affect health!

Persistent Organic Pollutants (POPs) are potentially toxic chemicals that are also known as "forever chemicals" because they are resistant to degradation through chemical, biological, and photolytic processes. They are almost impossible to detox both from the environment and the body! Hence the nickname "Forever chemicals". Plastic and Teflon, both fall into this group.

"Forever chemicals," are more formally known as per- and polyfluoroalkyl substances (PFAS) and have gained notoriety due to their persistence and potential harm to human health.

As a specific example, there are numerous chemicals that directly affect thyroid function, including (but not limited to):

Fluoride & fluorinated chemicals - fluoride is covered in detail in the heavy metal references.

PCB's or polychlorinated biphenyls - although the manufacture of these was banned in 1979 due to their harmful effects on human and environmental health, they still exist in the environment. PCBs can still be released to the environment from hazardous waste sites, illegal or improper disposal and can still affect health.

Flame retardants - which are used on furniture and electronics, as well as building materials to help prevent fires

Perchlorate - Manufactured perchlorate is used as an industrial chemical and can be found in rocket propellant, explosives, fireworks, and road flares, but is also used as an anti-static agent in food packaging. Perchlorate is both naturally occurring and a man-made contaminant that is increasingly found in groundwater, surface water, and soil. It is also used as a component in certain containers and food processing equipment for use in contact only with certain types of dry foods.

Bisphenol A (BPA) and other by-products of plastic - Primarily used in plastics, BPA is found in various products, including shatterproof windows, eyewear, water bottles, and epoxy resins that coat some metal food cans, bottle tops, and water supply pipes. Heat-printed receipts, like the ones we get from credit card transactions, all also major sources of BPA. It has a very similar shape to oestrogen and can bind to the same receptors, so along with affecting the thyroid, oestrogen-related health concerns are common. Oh, just so you are aware, BPA-free plastics still have other plastic compounds in them that are also potentially toxic, so BPA-free may not be as good as we thought it was.

Phthalates - Phthalates aren't one chemical; they are a CLASS of chemicals. Some types of phthalates are used in plastics, and some are used as a component of fragrances. They're found in many types of plastics, in food (due to food packaging and manufacturing equipment made of plastics), in household cleaners, personal care products, makeup, laundry products, pharmaceuticals, hospital equipment like tubing and blood bags, raincoats, clothing, wires and cables, and more.

Phthalate exposure doesn't only affect the thyroid, they have also been associated with:

- Allergy
- Asthma
- Type II diabetes and insulin resistance
- Overweight/obesity
- Reproductive issues in men and women

Because of how common these chemicals are - used in tens of thousands of products, exposure is also inevitable! While we can't ever avoid all exposure, we CAN work to minimise exposure in as many places as possible... in other words, we do what we can to reduce exposure.

To compound things, plastic is a massive stressor for the glucuronidation pathway, which we need to actively detox mould and mycotoxins. It is estimated that we consume, on average, a credit card's worth of plastic every single week. Every year, 52 credit cards worth of plastic gets into our bodies from the foods we eat, the air we breathe, and the water we drink every day. It is broken down into small enough particulates that we are even breathing it in when breathing in dirty air. There is a growing theory that mould has become more toxic over the past few years, due to climate change. But people are struggling more with it than they used to, and it is building up to higher levels. It is also not being cleared as readily. Is it, maybe, that we are being exposed to 52 credit cards worth of plastic every single year, stressing and depleting our glucuronidation pathway making the mouldiness worse?

Pollutants also have a very direct effect on the thyroid gland. With some form of thyroid disease being more prevalent than ever before, with women being 5-8 times more likely than men to develop thyroid dysfunction, it's important for people to be more aware of the toxins in their environment.

While there are specific compounds that seem to target the thyroid, others that impact gut health, and others that affect the neurological system, it's far easier from a practical perspective to just make reductions across the board than focus chemical by chemical.

These toxic compounds are found in various everyday products, including non-stick cookware, water-resistant fabrics, and firefighting foams. They're also used in thousands of industrial, medical, and military applications.

PFAS have been linked to an array of health issues, including cancer, reproductive disorders, and immune system dysfunction.

POPs are substances that remain intact for exceptionally long periods of time (many years), become widely distributed throughout the environment because of natural processes involving soil, water, and air, and bioaccumulate in the fatty tissue of living organisms.

They can be transported by wind and water, and most POPs generated in one country can and do affect people and wildlife far from where they are used and released. The most encountered POPs are organochlorine pesticides, such as DDT, industrial chemicals, polychlorinated biphenyls (PCB), as well as unintentional by-products of many industrial processes, especially polychlorinated dibenzo-p-dioxins (PCDD) and dibenzofurans (PCDF), commonly known as dioxins.

They are widely recognised, worldwide as being a risk to human health.

As they are so difficult to detox, focus on Phase 0 - remove the source! Then, support the basics and especially support glucuronidation.

- Don't walk around in your house with the same shoes you wear outside
- Stop buying scented candles and air fresheners
- Make sure your home or works paces are well ventilated
- Regularly wet dust and vacuum
- Assess the products you use on your skin, that you use to clean your house, and that are potentially in your environment, burdening you daily.
- Use glass or stainless steel, not plastic - and NEVER heat the plastic if you do use it.
- Eat clean - eat organic where possible
- Drink clean - filter your water (all of it, not just the water you drink)
- Breathe clean - get air purifiers
- Ensure phase 3 detoxification is effective
- Sweat - that will at least remove other toxins that may be burdening you
- Support Phase 2 detoxification as per the instructions in the book
- Bind - that will at least remove other toxins that may be burdening you

Chapter 22: Toxic People

Yes, you read that correctly; people can also be toxic! A toxic relationship is one that makes you feel unsupported, misunderstood, demeaned, or attacked and where your well-being is threatened in some way, whether emotionally, psychologically, or physically.

While every relationship goes through ups and downs, a toxic relationship is consistently unpleasant and draining for the people in it, to the point that negative moments outweigh and outnumber the positive ones.

Please note that a toxic relationship can be with a partner, child, friend or even your work environment, so please consider all of those when assessing whether you indeed have a toxic relationship in your life.

Here are some signs that you may be in a toxic relationship:

Feeling unsupported: A person in a toxic relationship may feel misunderstood and undermined in their relationship and may not feel encouraged to achieve their goals. A toxic person may see every achievement of the other person as a competition and will always try to one-up them.

Disrespectful behaviour: If there is a continuous pattern of selfish, negative, and disrespectful behaviour, then this may indicate that the relationship is toxic.

Lack of support: Relationships can become very negative if there is a lack of support from one or both sides. A person in a toxic relationship may feel unsupported and may not feel encouraged to achieve their goals.

Demeaning behaviour: A toxic partner may engage in demeaning behaviour, such as name-calling or belittling.

Controlling behaviour: A toxic partner may try to control the other person's behaviour, such as by dictating who they can see or what they can wear.

Dishonesty: A toxic partner may lie or withhold information from the other person.

Dominance: A toxic partner may try to dominate the other person, such as by making all the decisions or always having to be right.

Lack of communication: In a toxic relationship, communication tends to be unhealthy and reactive, with both partners avoiding taking any blame and ownership of their part in the conflict.

If you are in a toxic relationship, it is important to seek help and support. This may involve talking to a therapist, reaching out to a support group, or confiding in a trusted friend or family member. Your partner should support your decisions to support yourself.

In fact, the patients that have the best outcomes in my practice have partners who not only support the process, but they participate, whether they need to or not!

And now for something potentially controversial - **your relationship with YOURSELF!** The words you use when you speak to yourself are powerful! The words we use when speaking to ourselves, also known as self-talk or inner dialogue, can significantly impact our mental and emotional well-being, which in turn can influence our physical health. Here are a few ways in which the words we use when speaking to ourselves can affect our health:

Emotional State: The words we use in our self-talk can shape our emotional state. Negative self-talk, characterised by self-criticism, harsh judgments, and pessimistic thoughts, can contribute to feelings of stress, anxiety, and depression. These negative emotions can have detrimental effects on our overall health, including increased cortisol levels, impaired immune function, and disrupted sleep. When you find yourself speaking badly about your body's ability to heal, lose weight, and be better... stop and change the dialogue. Be grateful that it has kept you alive even through tremendous exposure to bad things; tell your body that you trust the process and LOVE yourself!

Stress Response: Negative self-talk can trigger the body's stress response, leading to the release of stress hormones such as cortisol and adrenaline. Prolonged or chronic activation of the stress response can have negative health consequences, including increased risk of cardiovascular disease, weakened immune system, and digestive issues. Stress can literally slow the process of healing down. I recommend a good cry, releasing those pent-up emotions, then working on stress management, meditation, walking in a forest, or even getting therapy.

Self-Perception and Self-Esteem: The way we speak to ourselves shapes our self-perception and self-esteem but also affects our ability to heal. Positive self-talk, characterised by self-encouragement, self-compassion, and affirmation, can enhance self-esteem and promote a healthier self-image. This positive self-perception can contribute to improved mental well-being and better overall health outcomes.

Behaviour and Motivation: The words we use when speaking to ourselves can influence our behaviours and motivation. Positive self-talk can foster self-belief, confidence, and motivation, encouraging us to engage in healthy behaviours such as exercise, proper nutrition, and self-care. On the other hand, negative self-talk can undermine motivation, leading to self-sabotage and unhealthy choices.

Perception of Pain and Illness: The words we use to describe pain or illness can impact our perception and experience of it. Research suggests that positive self-talk and reframing the way we think about pain can reduce pain intensity and improve coping mechanisms. Similarly, adopting a positive mindset and using empowering language when dealing with illness can contribute to a more proactive and resilient approach to healing.

It's important to be mindful of our self-talk and strive to cultivate positive, supportive inner dialogue. Practising self-awareness, self-compassion, and positive affirmations can help promote a healthier mindset and contribute to overall well-being. If negative self-talk persists or significantly impacts your mental or physical health, it may be beneficial to seek support from a mental health professional who can provide guidance and therapeutic interventions. One task I get some of my patients to do is to stand in front of a mirror (ideally naked, but that can be tough for some people in the beginning) and repeat to themselves:

I love you; I love you; I love you!

You can add other affirming statements like:

I am worthy, I am strong, I trust my body, etc.

This often results in tears, but eventually, something shifts, and healing is achieved! Finally, just a reminder that gut and brain health are not 2 separate things as previously thought! The current research in the worlds of psychology, neuroscience, nutrition, and gastroenterology supports my experience that improving gut health improves mental health and vice versa.

It is now widely accepted that many people with mental health conditions display brain inflammation at a cellular level. In other words when you experience periods of stress, anxiety, or depression it is likely you have increased inflammatory processes going on in your brain and body. To put simply, poor mental health is in part a state of inflammation.

We also know from research that gastric symptoms are linked to inflammation and a lack of diversity within the microbiome (which is like the guts eco-system). The more varied and diverse the microbiome is, the healthier the gut functions.

Interestingly we also know that many people with mental health symptoms have a lack of diversity with their gut microbiome. When this is treated (by feeding microbiome and encourage good bacteria to populate) mental health symptoms improve. It is believed that the increase in microbiome reduces inflammation which in turn improves mental health symptoms.

There are however a few other factors worth noting. The gut and brain are a two-way street in which information is transmitting back and forward all the time. The enteric nervous system and vagus nerve play crucial roles in ensuring information can be passed back and forward. If the gut is healthy, information tends to get through more easily. Think of it like creating a clear passage to enable fluid communication.

If the mind is healthy and less inflamed, this reduces sympathetic nervous responses that ordinarily aggravate the gut to prepare for fight, flight or freeze in times of stress or anxiety. Stress in many studies has been linked to aggravating gastrointestinal symptoms.

So, a healthy gut, supports a healthy mind. A healthy mind equally supports a healthy gut. The two are synonymous with each other. Therefore, harmony is vital.

It surprises me that many mental health treatments both therapeutically and pharmacologically still focus on the brain as a focal point of treatment. It is well documented that around 90% of serotonin and 50% of Dopamine is found in the lining of the gastrointestinal tract. These are just two of the chemicals associated with mood regulation and feeling 'good.'

The conversation needs to change but you can get started today on improving simultaneously your gut and mental health.

Chapter 23: Still Got Chemical Sensitivities?

If you still suffer from severe chemical sensitivities brought on by exposure to mould or pollutants, there is help in the form of DNRS. DNRS stands for Dynamic Neural Retraining System. It is a neuroplasticity-based therapy program designed to address chronic illnesses and sensitivities, including conditions like multiple chemical sensitivities (MCS), chronic fatigue syndrome (CFS), fibromyalgia, and other related conditions. The DNRS program was developed by Annie Hopper, who experienced severe environmental sensitivities herself. There is another DNRS program called the Gupta Method; either one can prove useful.

The underlying principle of DNRS is based on the concept of neuroplasticity, which refers to the brain's ability to rewire and create new neural pathways. The program aims to rewire the brain's response to perceived threats, helping individuals regain health and reduce sensitivities.

DNRS focuses on retraining the limbic system, which is the part of the brain responsible for emotional and behavioural responses, including the fight-or-flight response. It aims to calm the hyperactive limbic system, which may contribute to sensitivities and symptoms.

It involves a series of specific exercises and techniques that aim to interrupt maladaptive neural patterns and help establish new, healthier patterns. These exercises involve visualisation, positive neuroplasticity exercises, and cognitive techniques to redirect the brain's responses. DNRS also emphasises the mind-body connection and the role of emotions and beliefs in health and healing. It addresses the impact of stress, trauma, and negative thought patterns on the body's sensitivities and overall well-being.

Through consistent practice and repetition, DNRS aims to reprogram the brain's responses to various triggers, reducing sensitivities and symptoms over time. This involves creating new neural connections and patterns that promote a sense of safety and well-being.

It's important to note that while some individuals report positive outcomes with DNRS, the scientific evidence supporting its effectiveness is limited. The program has gained popularity among some individuals with sensitivities, but it may not be suitable or effective for everyone.

If you are considering DNRS or seeking treatment for sensitivities, it's advisable to consult with a healthcare professional who specialises in the specific condition you're dealing with. They can provide guidance, personalised recommendations, and evidence-based treatments that align with your individual needs and circumstances.

Scan the QR code if you want to try the Gupta program:

Chapter 24: Hormones - How They Are Affected by Bad Stuff

In my experience, one of the first symptoms people will notice when they are affected by heavy metals, mould, pollutants or a toxic relationship, is a change in their hormones. In this chapter I will give some basic guidance on hormones and how to best test them and to balance them using good things BUT, I will need to write another book to fully explain this, or you could find another book to guide you further. Hormones are tiny, complicated, yet simple, chemical messengers that are very affected by exposure to bad things! Any change in hormones should be investigated as soon as possible by a qualified healthcare provider!

The 3 sets of hormones I am going to cover very briefly in this chapter are often referred to as the "sisters" because they are so closely related that when 1 is affected, the others are also affected.

They are: The thyroid (energy), the adrenal glands (stress) and the sex hormones (joy). There are many other hormones, but these are considerably more affected by toxins. Although I am touching on a very complex topic, should you find any imbalances in any tests you do, please take professional medical advice!

Thyroid (energy):

The thyroid is specifically sensitive to toxins and imbalances. I have mentioned it a few times already. It is so sensitive that it is referred to as "the canary in the coal mine" and people will often have signs and symptoms of an under or overactive thyroid when they have nutritional imbalances. They will often get the relevant treatment for the symptoms but not get any better. That is because the root cause of the canary dying, isn't that the canary is sick, but that it is being poisoned by its environment (the mine)!

When someone presents with thyroid symptoms, I will absolutely run a thyroid function test, but I will also run a toxic metal panel to assess the other things that affect thyroid function, such as bromine (same family as iodine but not the same function), arsenic and mercury. The test also assesses selenium, iodine and the other nutrients the thyroid needs to function properly Thyroid hormones are best assessed via a blood test. I use both serum and dried blood spot tests (not both at the same time, one or the other), depending on the case.

Levels of key thyroid hormones can indicate whether there is a thyroid imbalance. These include:

TSH - Produced by the pituitary gland, TSH acts on the thyroid gland to stimulate production of the thyroid hormone thyroxine (T4).

Free T4 – Thyroxine - The predominant hormone produced by the thyroid gland, T4 is converted to its active form, T3, within cells using selenium and Iron. It is made up of 4 Iodine molecules.

Total T4 – Thyroxine - Total T4 includes both free T4 and protein-bound T4 and is an indicator of the thyroid gland's ability to synthesise, process and release T4 into the bloodstream.

Free T3 – Triiodothyronine - T3 is the active thyroid hormone that regulates the metabolic activity of cells.

TPOab – Thyroid Peroxidase Antibodies - Thyroid peroxidase is an enzyme involved in thyroid hormone production. The body produces antibodies, including TPOab, that attack the thyroid gland in autoimmune thyroiditis and Hashimoto's. Testing TPOab levels can diagnose these conditions.

Tgbn – Thyroglobulin - A protein rich in tyrosine, the residues of which when bound to iodine become the building blocks of T3 and T4. If iodine levels are low, thyroglobulin accumulates, thus high levels indicate insufficient iodine for healthy thyroid function.

If I suspect the adrenals are very involved, and the levels of T3 and T4 seem normal on an initial test, I will run a Reverse T3 (RT3) test. The stress hormone cortisol increases conversion of T4 into reverse T3 hence why the adrenals should be assessed. Other factors to consider if RT3 is high is blood sugar imbalances, inflammation or poor nutrition.

Hyperthyroidism symptoms include:

Weight loss

Increased appetite

Fast heart rate

Anxiety/nervousness

Irritability

Shaking/trembling of the hands

Sweating

Feeling warm often/greater sensitivity to heat

Insomnia

Frequent bowel movements and/or diarrhoea

Muscle weakness

Thin skin and brittle hair

Changes in the menstrual cycle (usually shorter, lighter periods)

Hypothyroidism symptoms include:

Weight gain and/or difficulty losing weight

Constipation

Fatigue

Forgetfulness

Depression

Dry skin and hair/hair loss

Slow heart rate

Feeling cold often/greater sensitivity to cold

Changes in the menstrual cycle (usually longer, heavier periods)

Adrenals (stress):

I also always assess adrenal health at the same time. Often addressing the adrenals, removing any offending metals and stressors and replacing the good stuff, will cause healing to occur without the need for any additional interventions.

The best way to assess the adrenals is to do both a salivary cortisol 4-point test (that means you do it at 4 specific times of the day) which would assess the free, unbound, active cortisol, along with a urinary metabolite test that assesses the total cortisol made as well as the inactive cortisone. From these 2 sample types you get a more accurate picture of the health of the adrenal glands. You can also assess DHEA and DHEAs in both blood and as urinary metabolites. DHEA is also considered a sex hormone and requires a specific balance. If you find an imbalance in a test, please consult with your healthcare provider as there are many supplements and medications that can help you treat the cause.

Signs and symptoms of adrenal insufficiency may include:

Fatigue(physical and mental)
Body aches
Unexplained weight loss/gain
Low blood pressure
Lightheadedness
Loss of body hair
Skin discolouration (hyperpigmentation)
A fatty lump between the shoulders.
Pink or purple stretch marks on the stomach, hips, thighs, breasts and underarms.
Thin, frail skin that bruises easily.
Slow wound healing.

Gonadal/sex (joy):

Then there are the gonadal/sex hormones. Although women will most likely notice a change before men do, it doesn't mean that men don't experience imbalances. In fact, quite the opposite is true, they experience mode changes, low libido, even breast cancer! They should also be assessed fully! I use blood and dried urine metabolite tests when assessing these hormones, to get a full picture of what the body is doing and how it is managing to detox them. There are a couple of very good labs that do the dried urine testing, but please don't do one without the guidance of a qualified professional who understands them, as they are often confusing if you don't know what all the markers mean!

Dehydroepiandrosterone (DHEA) is a hormone that your body naturally produces in the adrenal gland. DHEA helps produce other hormones, including testosterone and oestrogen. Natural DHEA levels peak in early adulthood and then slowly fall as you age. DHEAs is made in the adrenal glands and converts to testosterone and androstenedione then oestrogen.

In men, testosterone is made in the testes, in women, testosterone is produced in various locations. One quarter of the hormone is produced in the ovary, a quarter is produced in the adrenal gland, and one half is produced in the peripheral tissues from the various precursors produced in the ovaries and adrenal gland. Testosterone is generally considered a male hormone but ask any menopausal woman about what made her libido come back after bio identical hormone replacement therapy (BHRT), most will say it was testosterone. Testosterone also brings back lagging energy levels. Low testosterone in both men and women is often related to stress. In men, there will be issues with erectile dysfunction and general low mood.

Testosterone can also be too high; this is usually more of an issue in women than in men. In some women this is normal, and they have no symptoms, such as male pattern hair loss or hair growth on the face, however, some women do have symptoms and should be properly assessed. The main nutrient linked to testosterone is zinc, so please assess zinc (and copper) if you see any imbalance. If testosterone is causing issues, you can balance it using premade formulas designed for prostate health. Yes, I know, women don't have prostates, but the formulas work on women in the same way they do in men, helping them to detox the hormone in a safer way.

Oestrogen can be affected by copper imbalances as well as a mycotoxin called Zearanolone and a POP called Bisphenol A, both of which have a very similar structure to oestrogen. Oestrogen can also get affected by the microbiome and the enzyme Beta-glucuronidase. So, if you see issues with oestrogen being too high, remember all these factors can influence this hormone. The ovaries don't make too much oestrogen, it is what happens afterwards, whether it can be detoxed through the liver properly and whether it moves out the body into the toilet, these are what usually make oestrogen dominant states.

Oestrogen too low may mean menopause, or a copper deficiency. Please remember to evaluate men for oestrogen issues as well, they are not immune to them! Low levels of sex hormones can also be due to stress. You can either be in your happy, parasympathetic nervous system, which allows you to feed and breed, rest and digest... or you can be in you sympathetic, fight, fright, flight nervous system. You can't be in both, so if you are very stressed, this will impact fertility!

Progesterone balances oestrogen. This hormone only appears after ovulation and should be in balance with oestrogen. Some people can also be progesterone dominant and get migraines and moodiness after ovulation that is often mistaken as oestrogen issues. Iron and progesterone have a specific relationship, so in cases where there is iron deficiency, usually from heavy bleeding, remember to assess progesterone as well as oestrogen, iron as well as copper. Progesterone is also affected by stress, so always assess the adrenal health if you see issues with progesterone.

There are many signs and symptoms to look out for but to simplify things, if you are a woman, ANY change in your cycle is something to note. ANY symptoms are a sign of imbalance, that would include but are not exclusive to:

Heavy bleeding
Changes in colour of menstrual blood
Period pain, no one should suffer!
Migraines
Weight gain

Moodiness
Brain fog
Growth of hair where you don't want
Loss of hair where you do want it!
If you are male:
Change in libido or sexual performance
Moodiness
Lack of energy

Hormones should be assessed alongside any potential toxicities! Hormonal imbalance are early signs that bad things are affecting you.

Chapter 25: A Guide to Using Food as Medicine

There are so many "healthy diets" these days, I am sure you are probably aware of them. I believe that if we simplify the rules, don't vilify anything that is a "real food", make sure there is good balance of nutrients, choose and chew your food well, then you are going to feel healthier anyway! There are easy recipes in the eBook on the website, that incorporate as many of the good things that support the body; feel free to try them, adapt them to your specific tastes, and stay healthy! Just 3 rules you should stick to:

1. If you can't eat it within 24 hours, either freeze it, or throw it away!
2. If your grandparent wouldn't call it food, don't eat it.
3. Source your food locally and seasonally where possible.

The basics are Proteins (that break down to amino acids that helps us the rebuild), Carbohydrates (that provide energy) and Fats (that provide energy and the basics for cell membranes and neurological health). I will also refer to "the rainbow" often, this will be the colourful vegetables and fruits that will supply healing nutrients. A variety of each, sourced locally, seasonally and fresh will be a great way to start your healing. I will also cover some excellent herbs, spice and mushrooms!

Finally, there are the fats. Fats can be excellent for your health, or they can harm you, so please choose wisely.

Protein:

This should be a priority at each meal. We need protein to repair, heal, and, most importantly, to detox. Proteins, primarily enzymes, are involved in all six phases 2 detoxification pathways to catalyse the conjugation reactions that render toxic substances more water-soluble and ready for elimination from the body.

The best sources of proteins are from animals (sorry vegetarians) but also some vegetables (yay).

Animal proteins - Animal protein sources are abundant and offer a range of nutrients. Here are some of the best sources of animal protein and some healthy cooking methods:

Wild or free-range Poultry: Chicken, duck, and turkey are excellent sources of protein rich animal protein. They can be grilled, baked, or sautéed with suitable added fats or oils. Avoid deep-frying or using highly processed sauces to keep the dish healthier.

Fish: Fatty fish, like salmon, mackerel, sardines, and trout are not only rich in protein but also provide omega-3 fatty acids. Baking, grilling, or steaming fish are healthy cooking methods that help retain nutrients. Avoid breading and deep-frying.

Eggs: Eggs are a versatile and nutrient-dense source of animal protein. They can be boiled, poached, or scrambled using minimal oil or butter. Avoid excessive overheating if frying.

Grass-fed Meat: All cuts of grass-fed beef, such as fillet, sirloin, tenderloin, are good sources of animal protein but please make sure they are grass fed. Lamb and venison tend to be free-range and grass-fed, so are also excellent choices. Also, they tend not to have too many added medications. Happy pigs, reared in a way that keeps them healthy and stress free, are also excellent sources of protein. Grilling, broiling, or slow roasting are healthier cooking methods.

Dairy Products: Unless you have issues with lactose and casein, dairy products like Greek yoghurt, cottage cheese, and whole milk provide protein along with calcium and other essential nutrients. These products are commonly consumed raw or incorporated into recipes.

Seafood: Shellfish such as shrimp, crab, and lobster are protein-rich options. Grilling, steaming, or boiling seafood can be healthier cooking methods. However, be mindful of added sauces or butter, as they can increase the calorie and trans-fat content. Also, be aware not to eat seafood a week before testing for heavy metals.

Vegetable sources of protein include nuts, legumes and even some vegetables. Here are some to consider including in your diet:

Nuts and seeds - There are many to choose from. Soak the nuts and seeds before use; just use a handful a day maximum.

Legumes: Legumes such as lentils, chickpeas, black beans, kidney beans, and soybeans are excellent sources of plant-based protein. They are versatile and can be used in various dishes like soups, stews, salads, and curries. Some people are quite reactive to legumes though, so if you find you are getting gassy and cramps, please eliminate these.

Quinoa: Quinoa is a seed that is often considered a grain and is a complete protein source, meaning it contains all essential amino acids. It is highly nutritious and can be used as a base for salads, side dishes, or even as a substitute for rice.

Tofu and Tempeh: Tofu and tempeh are soy-based products that are rich in protein. They are commonly used in vegetarian and vegan cooking as meat substitutes. Tofu has a mild flavour and can be cooked in various ways, such as stir-frying, grilling, or blending into smoothies. Tempeh has a firmer texture and nuttier flavour and can be marinated and grilled, used in stir-fries, or crumbled into sauces and stews.

Edamame: Edamame is young soybeans that are harvested before they harden. They are commonly boiled or steamed and can be enjoyed as a snack or added to salads, stir-fries, or rice dishes.

Chia Seeds: Chia seeds are a great source of plant-based protein, along with healthy fats and fibre. They can be added to smoothies, yoghurt, or oatmeal, or used as an egg substitute in baking recipes.

Green Peas: Green peas are not only rich in protein but also provide fibre and various vitamins and minerals. They can be added to salads, stir-fries, soups, or served as a side dish.

Spirulina: Spirulina is a type of blue-green algae that is rich in protein and contains all essential amino acids. It is available in powder or tablet form and can be added to smoothies or used as a supplement.

Remember, while these vegetable sources of protein are beneficial, it's essential to have a varied diet to ensure you get a complete range of essential amino acids. Combining different plant-based protein sources throughout the day can help you achieve a balanced protein intake. Some of these plant-based proteins are also a source of carbohydrates.

Protein digestion occurs primarily in the mouth, from chewing, then in the stomach, where the acid and enzymes break the protein into the base molecule's amino acids. It is important to make sure your stomach is acidic enough to do this. Regulating stress, chewing your food well, and being mindful when eating can all help. If needed, you can use bitter herbs to stimulate gastric fluids to further improve digestion.

When it comes to aiding protein digestion, there are several bitter herbs that can be beneficial. Bitter herbs help stimulate digestive function by promoting the production of digestive enzymes and enhancing overall digestive health. Here are a few bitter herbs that are commonly used to support protein digestion:

Dandelion (Taraxacum officinale): Dandelion leaves and roots are known for their bitter taste. They can stimulate the production of digestive enzymes, including proteases that help break down proteins.

Gentian (Gentiana lutea): Gentian root is one of the most potent bitter herbs available. It stimulates the production of saliva, gastric juices, and bile, which aids in the digestion of proteins.

Artichoke (Cynara scolymus): Artichoke contains a compound called cynarin, which has bitter properties. It promotes bile flow and aids in the digestion of fats and proteins.

Wormwood (Artemisia absinthium): Wormwood is a bitter herb traditionally used as a digestive tonic. It can help stimulate appetite and support the digestion of proteins.

Gentianella (Gentianella alborosea): This herb belongs to the same family as gentian and shares similar bitter properties. It can stimulate digestive secretions and improve protein digestion.

Milk thistle (Silybum marianum): Although primarily known for its liver-protective properties, milk thistle also has a bitter taste. It stimulates bile production, which aids in the digestion of fats and proteins.

It's important to note that individual responses to bitter herbs may vary, and it's advisable to consult a healthcare professional or a qualified herbalist before incorporating them into your routine, especially if you have any underlying health conditions or are taking medications.

Carbohydrates:

Although some people believe all carbohydrates are bad, that is not true of naturally occurring carbs found in fruit and vegetables. The best carbs come in the form of vegetables, with fruit as an occasional treat. Vegetables contain colours called phytonutrients, which play a crucial role in supporting the body's natural detoxification processes. Vegetables provide various nutrients and compounds that aid in detoxification in the following ways:

Antioxidants: Vegetables are rich in antioxidants, including vitamins C and E, beta-carotene, and various phytochemicals. These compounds help neutralise harmful free radicals and protect cells from damage caused by toxins and oxidative stress.

Fibre: Many vegetables are excellent sources of dietary fibre. Fibre acts as a natural cleanser for the digestive system by promoting regular bowel movements and preventing constipation. It helps bind toxins, cholesterol, and waste products, aiding their elimination from the body.

Water content: Vegetables, particularly leafy greens and watery vegetables like cucumbers and celery, have high water content. Staying hydrated is important for optimal detoxification as it supports kidney function, which is crucial for filtering waste and toxins from the blood.

Chlorophyll: Leafy green vegetables like spinach, and parsley are rich in chlorophyll, a pigment responsible for their green colour. Chlorophyll has been found to aid in the elimination of toxins and heavy metals from the body by binding to them and promoting their excretion.

Phytonutrients: Vegetables contain a wide array of phytonutrients, including flavonoids, polyphenols, and sulphur compounds. These bioactive compounds have been shown to support detoxification processes, including the activation of enzymes involved in phase 1 and phase 2 detox pathways.

However; some vegetables can also contain things called "anti-nutrients" that stop you from getting the benefits of the good stuff. Thankfully there are ways to reduce these, so you get more benefits. Here are some of the ways to reduce the potential anti-nutrients:

- **Sprouting** - soak your seeds and wait for them to sprout. The best sprouts for detoxification are broccoli sprouts but all sprouts have some benefit so eat a variety.

- **Soaking** (adding lactic acid bacteria, diluted hydrogen peroxide, iodine, vinegar, or baking soda to the soaking water may boost the soaking process e.g., for removal of phytates).
- **Boiling or blanching** (reduces oxalate levels, etc.)
- **Cooking** (significantly reduces lectin and oxalate levels)
- **Lactic acid fermentation** (significantly reduces phytotoxins in cassava and phytic acid in cereal products).

Although there are benefits from the full rainbow of colourful vegetables and you should aim to get a variety into you, change them up regularly to get even more benefits!

Liver-supporting vegetables to focus on:

Cruciferous vegetables: These include broccoli, cabbage, brussels sprouts, contain compounds like glucosinolates that support liver function and enhance the production of enzymes involved in detoxification pathways.

Leafy Greens: Leafy greens such as spinach, kale, Swiss chard, and collard greens are nutrient-dense and rich in chlorophyll. They help eliminate toxins and support liver function. These greens are also excellent sources of antioxidants, vitamins, and minerals. Some leafy greens, such as spinach and kale, can contain oxalates and are best blanched rather than raw.

Garlic and Onions: Garlic and onions are known for their sulphur-containing compounds, such as allicin, which support liver function and assist in the detoxification process. They also provide antioxidants and have antimicrobial properties.

Artichokes: Artichokes contain a compound called cynarin, which supports liver function and promotes bile production. Bile plays a crucial role in eliminating toxins from the liver and aiding digestion.

Beets: Beets are rich in antioxidants and contain compounds such as betaine and betalains that support liver function. They aid in the body's natural detoxification processes and help purify the blood.

Carrots: Carrots are rich in antioxidants, particularly beta-carotene, which supports liver health. They also provide fibre and assist in promoting regular bowel movements for the efficient elimination of waste and toxins.

Coriander/Cilantro: Cilantro, also known as coriander leaves, is an herb with detoxifying properties. It contains compounds that aid in the elimination of heavy metals from the body.

Dandelion Greens: Dandelion greens have been traditionally used to support liver health and stimulate bile production. They are rich in antioxidants and nutrients that aid in detoxification.

As mentioned before, fruits should be limited to reduce the sugar load while detoxing, but small portions in salads and combined into meals can still be beneficial and can be a treat.

Here are some fruits known for their detoxification-supporting properties:

Citrus Fruits: Citrus fruits like lemons, limes, oranges, and grapefruits are rich in vitamin C, which is an antioxidant that helps neutralise toxins and supports liver function. They also contain flavonoids and limonoids that aid in detoxification. Use the zest as well as the fruit to get the most benefit.

Berries: Berries, such as blueberries, strawberries, raspberries, and blackberries, are packed with antioxidants, including anthocyanins. These antioxidants help protect cells from damage caused by toxins and oxidative stress.

Apples: Apples are high in fibre, particularly pectin, which can help eliminate toxins and heavy metals from the body. They also provide antioxidants and support digestive health.

Pineapple: Pineapple contains an enzyme called bromelain, which aids in digestion and has anti-inflammatory properties. It supports the body's natural detoxification processes by promoting healthy digestion.

Pomegranate: Pomegranates are rich in antioxidants, particularly punicalagin, which have been shown to have protective effects on the liver. Pomegranate juice or seeds can be consumed to support detoxification.

Watermelon: Watermelon is hydrating and has a high-water content, which supports kidney function and helps flush out toxins. It also contains the antioxidant lycopene, which has been linked to liver health.

Papaya: Papaya contains an enzyme called papain, which aids in digestion and supports the breakdown of proteins. It also provides fibre and antioxidants that assist in detoxification.

Kiwi: Kiwi is packed with vitamin C and fibre, which support immune function and digestive health. It provides antioxidants that help protect against oxidative stress and aid in detoxification.

Incorporating a variety of these fruits into your diet can provide essential nutrients and antioxidants that support the body's natural detoxification processes. Enjoy them as whole fruits, add them to smoothies, or incorporate them into salads for a nutritious and detox-friendly meal.

Teas. Certain teas are known for their potential detoxification-supporting properties. They can also provide hydration, antioxidants, and potentially beneficial compounds.

Here are some teas often associated with detoxification:

Green Tea: Green tea is rich in antioxidants called catechins, particularly epigallocatechin gallate (EGCG). These compounds have been studied for their potential health benefits, including supporting liver function and aiding in the body's natural detoxification processes.

Dandelion Tea: Dandelion tea is derived from the leaves or roots of the dandelion plant. It is believed to have diuretic properties, which may help promote urine production and assist in flushing out toxins from the body. Dandelion tea is also commonly used to support liver health.

Milk Thistle Tea: Milk thistle tea is made from the seeds of the milk thistle plant. It contains a flavonoid called silymarin, which is believed to have liver-protective properties and support the liver's detoxification processes.

Ginger Tea: Ginger tea has been traditionally used for its digestive properties. It may support digestion, reduce inflammation, and potentially aid in detoxification by promoting healthy digestion and elimination.

Peppermint Tea: Peppermint tea is known for its soothing properties on the digestive system. It may help relieve bloating, support healthy digestion, and promote the elimination of waste products.

Rooibos Tea: Rooibos tea is an herbal tea derived from the leaves of the Aspalathus linearis plant. It is rich in antioxidants and may have anti-inflammatory properties. While research specifically on its detoxification effects is limited, its antioxidant content can support overall health.

Nettle Tea: Nettle tea is made from the leaves and roots of the nettle plant. It is believed to have diuretic properties and may support kidney function and fluid balance. By promoting urine production, it may assist in eliminating toxins from the body.

Liquorice tea: Liquorice root is rich in antioxidants, which help protect the body's cells from damage caused by free radicals. Antioxidants play a role in supporting overall health and may contribute to the body's natural detoxification processes. Potential Considerations: While liquorice tea can be enjoyed in moderation, it's important to note that excessive consumption or prolonged use of liquorice root can have potential side effects. Liquorice root contains a compound called glycyrrhizin, which can lead to increased blood pressure and lower potassium levels in some individuals. It's advisable to consult with a healthcare professional, especially if you have any underlying health conditions or are taking medications.

There are many others, like hibiscus and even black tea, in moderation. I recommend trying a range and finding the ones you like the most, then drinking a variety of those regularly.

As always, it's recommended to consult with a healthcare professional before making significant changes to your diet or incorporating new herbal teas, especially if you have specific health concerns or conditions.

Then there are the delicious herbs and spices that not only make your food taste amazing, but they also help various biological processes, and you should try and include them in more dishes. Several herbs & spices can be consumed as part of a balanced diet to support the body's natural detoxification processes.

Here are some herbs known for their potential detoxification-supporting properties:

Burdock Root: Burdock root has been traditionally used in herbal medicine for its potential detoxifying and blood-purifying properties. It can be consumed cooked or in herbal tea form.

Turmeric: Turmeric is a vibrant yellow spice commonly used in cooking. It contains a compound called curcumin, which has anti-inflammatory properties and supports liver health. Adding turmeric to dishes or consuming it as a tea can contribute to detoxification support.

Mustard: Addition of raw or slightly cooked mustard seeds to cooked brassica provides a natural source of myrosinase enzyme needed to convert glucoraphanin to sulforaphane.

Ginger: Ginger is a versatile herb used for its potential digestive benefits. It can help support healthy digestion, reduce inflammation, and aid in detoxification processes.

Peppermint: Peppermint leaves are often used to make herbal tea. Peppermint tea can support digestion, relieve bloating, and promote the elimination of waste products.

Parsley: Parsley is a common culinary herb rich in antioxidants, vitamins, and minerals. It can support liver health and aid in the body's natural detoxification processes.

Cinnamon: This delicious spice can improve cholesterol as well as balance blood sugar

Rosemary - Rosemary contains a strong antioxidant called carnosol, which can help detoxify and balance hormones, specifically oestrogen.

Medical mushrooms - Some people say you should avoid mushrooms if you are mouldy; I have, however, seen benefits that outweigh any concerns!

Medical mushrooms, also known functional mushrooms, are a group of mushrooms that have been traditionally used in various cultures for their potential health benefits. They are rich in bioactive compounds, including polysaccharides, beta-glucans, triterpenes, and antioxidants, which contribute to their therapeutic properties. Medical mushrooms have been associated with several health benefits that can support overall well-being. Here are some ways medical mushrooms may contribute to health:

Immune Support: Many medical mushrooms, such as Reishi (Ganoderma lucidum), Turkey Tail (Trametes versicolor), and Cordyceps (Cordyceps sinensis) and shiitake have been studied for their potential immune-modulating properties. They may help support a healthy immune system, which plays a crucial role in detoxification processes.

Anti-Inflammatory Effects: Medical mushrooms contain compounds that possess anti-inflammatory properties. Chronic inflammation can contribute to various health issues, so reducing inflammation can promote overall well-being.

Antioxidant Activity: Medical mushrooms are rich in antioxidants, such as phenols and polysaccharides, which help neutralise free radicals and protect cells from oxidative damage. Antioxidants support overall health and may contribute to the body's natural detoxification processes.

Liver Support: Some medical mushrooms, including Reishi and Turkey Tail, have been studied for their potential hepatoprotective effects. They may support liver health and aid in the liver's detoxification processes.

Adaptogenic Properties: Certain medical mushrooms, such as Reishi and Cordyceps, are classified as adaptogens. Adaptogens help the body adapt to stress, promote balance, and support overall well-being.

It's recommended to source medical mushrooms from reputable suppliers to ensure their quality and safety.

Here are some common culinary mushrooms that offer nutritional benefits:

Shiitake Mushrooms: Shiitake mushrooms are known for their savoury flavour and are rich in vitamins, minerals, and dietary fibre. They contain compounds like beta-glucans that have been studied for their potential immune-enhancing properties.

Portobello Mushrooms: Portobello mushrooms are a larger, mature version of cremini mushrooms. They are a good source of B vitamins, potassium, and dietary fibre. Portobello mushrooms are often used as a meat substitute due to their hearty texture.

Maitake Mushrooms: Maitake mushrooms have a unique, frilly shape and a rich flavour. They contain various nutrients, including B vitamins, minerals, and polysaccharides that may support immune function.

White Button Mushrooms: White button mushrooms are the most widely available and commonly consumed mushrooms. They are low in calories and provide nutrients such as B vitamins, selenium, and potassium.

Oyster Mushrooms: Oyster mushrooms have a delicate flavour and are often used in Asian cuisine. They are a good source of protein, B vitamins, and minerals such as potassium and phosphorus. They can even down-regulate an enzyme called Aromatase that converts testosterone into oestrogen.

Enoki Mushrooms: Enoki mushrooms have long, thin stems and a mild flavour. They are low in calories and contain nutrients like B vitamins, fibre, and potassium.

Cremini Mushrooms: Cremini mushrooms are often referred to as baby portobellos and have a slightly stronger flavour compared to white button mushrooms. They provide nutrients such as B vitamins, selenium, and potassium.

It's important to note that while culinary mushrooms offer nutritional value, they should be consumed as part of a balanced diet that includes a variety of fruits, vegetables, whole grains, and other nutrient-rich foods. Maintaining a healthy lifestyle overall, including regular exercise, proper hydration, and adequate sleep, is also important for supporting the body's natural detoxification processes.

Fats:

When I was younger, fats were demonised, and the trend was for everything to be fat free. What we saw as a result was an increase in skin issues, mental health issues and an overall reduction, not in increase, in the health of the general population. Also, weirdly enough, people were also getting fatter! Over time, fats have become recognised as being vital for healing. It is now almost common knowledge to understand that Omega 3 has anti-inflammatory effects on the body.

Healthy fats play a crucial role in maintaining good health. They offer various benefits, including supporting heart health, brain function, and overall well-being. Here's a list of healthy fats, their benefits, and some common sources:

Monounsaturated fats: They can help reduce bad LDL cholesterol levels and lower the risk of heart disease. Best sources are Olive oil, Avocados, Nuts (almonds, cashews, peanuts), Seeds (flaxseeds, chia seeds), Nut butters (almond butter, peanut butter)

Polyunsaturated fat: These fats are essential for brain function and have anti-inflammatory properties. They can also help lower LDL cholesterol. Best sources include Fatty fish (salmon, trout, mackerel), Flaxseeds and flaxseed oil, Walnuts, Sunflower seeds (not sunflower oil though)

Omega 3: They are known to support heart and brain health, reduce inflammation, and may help with depression and anxiety. Best sources include Grass fed meats, Fatty fish (salmon, sardines, tuna), Chia seeds, Flaxseeds, Walnuts, Hemp seeds & Algal oil (for vegetarians and vegans).

Omega 6: Although often vilified as an inflammatory oil, some omega 6 is also beneficial. Along with omega-3 fatty acids, omega-6 fatty acids play a crucial role in brain function, and normal growth and development. As a type of polyunsaturated fatty acid (PUFA), omega-6s help stimulate skin and hair growth, maintain bone health, regulate metabolism, and maintain the reproductive system. Good sources include walnuts, safflower oil, tofu, hemp and sunflower seeds.

Omega 7: This comes from Sea Buckthorn Berry Oil and is amazing for skin conditions and can even help women who have post-menopausal vaginal dryness, as it mostly supports maintenance of normal mucous membranes and skin

Omega 9: This can help improve blood sugar control and reduce inflammation. Best sources include, olive oil, avocado oil, macadamia nuts and almonds.

Medium chain triglycerides: MCTs are rapidly absorbed and can be used for quick energy. They may aid in weight management and support brain function. Best sources include Coconut oil, Palm kernel oil, MCT oil supplements.

General dietary Recommendations (more specific ones are in the next section)

Eat as your ancestors would, choose grass-fed meat options, wild oily fish with a side of veg, and low to no grains. Prepare a diet low in farmed animal proteins (organic and grass-fed are OK) and refined carbohydrates and high in potassium-rich fruits and vegetables. This regimen maintains the body's stores of calcium, potassium, and magnesium and promotes urinary excretion of oestrogen-like compounds. Ask yourself, "would my great grandparents recognise this as food", if the answer is no, then maybe consider another option. Here are some more guidelines to eating a healthy diet:

- Only eat freshly prepared food, no leftovers.
- Emphasise organic, natural whole foods to minimise exposure to antibiotics, hormones, pesticides, artificial colours/flavours/sugars, high fructose corn syrup, or preservatives.
- Consume a variety of vegetables and fruits.
- Adequate fluid intake facilitates the action of fibre. A minimum of 100ml filtered water eight times per day is recommended.
- Kefir 50-100ml can help mould and gut health.
- Have small amounts of gluten-free grains, if tolerated: Quinoa, brown rice, wild rice, oats.

Note that grains, even organic and gluten-free, are still likely to harbour some level of mould of mycotoxins simply due to the methods by which they are stored and processed. It may require some self-experimentation to determine whether you can tolerate any grains in your low-mould diet.

If you have MOULD allergies - AVOID where possible or eat in small amounts only:

- Leftovers of any kind but especially cooked rice (If you are eating rice, eat it within 24 hours of cooking it, then discard!
- All types of cheese - for a while, at least
- Nuts and seeds - for a while at least. Peanuts are especially known to be very prone to mould.
- Vinegar and foods preserved in vinegar: Salad dressings, mustard, olives, white vinegar - this includes apple cider vinegar.
- Sour cream, sour milk, buttermilk, yogurt - except kefir
- Alcoholic beverages: Beer, wine (you can have whiskey, Gin or Vodka in moderation)
- Sourdough bread
- Sauerkraut and other fermented vegetables

- Preserved meats: smoked meats, smoked fish, sausages, corned beef, ham, bacon
- Non-grass-fed meat can also contain mycotoxins from the grains they were fed.
- All dried fruits: Raisins, apricots, cranberries, figs, prunes
- Canned juice
- Canned tomatoes
- Corn
- High-sugar foods and processed foods should be avoided, as sugar will feed the fungal infection.
- Pineapple, melons, and citrus have a higher propensity for developing mould.
- Honeydew melon and cantaloupe are two prime examples; you can often see mould growing directly on the rind of these melons (unless a toxic fungicide has been applied, but it would be best to avoid that too!)
- You may want to avoid eating canned foods, even if those foods are not on the "mould-containing foods" list. If any mould spores enter a vat of food before it is divided up and canned, the spores can replicate in the can to a degree significant enough to cause illness.
- Coffee can contain mould spores; consider purchasing a mould-free brand of coffee; these are available online.

Wash and peel fruits and vegetables that have grown from the ground before eating. Mould is present in the soil and can contaminate the skins of fruits and vegetables.

Other things that help after you have cleaned up your food choices:

- Dry brush and rebound to stimulate lymph flow
- Infrared sauna or sauna blanket - either will help
- Epsom salts baths - add 1-2 cups of epsom salts to your hot bath and add some aromatherapy oils to help you relax; you can even add thyme, oregano, clove etc. for the mould
- Air purifiers and dehumidifiers
- Water filters - anything is better than nothing!

- And if you need it - Practising the Gupta method or DNRS

Get the basics covered:

Get the BAD STUFF out:

Use the free tools to assess yourself and reassess every three months
Support detoxification through food and supplements, use appropriate binders
Sweat (Sauna)
Poop and pee
Assess your relationships
Get tested and address that specific toxic burden.
Work with a functional medicine doctor.

Get the GOOD STUFF in:

Eat clean, prioritise protein, good fats, and organic rainbow plants, go gluten low
Chew your food more than you think you should
Drink clean filtered water and plenty of it
Breathe clean by using air purifiers
Sleep
Move
Lymph drainage
Epsom salts baths
Red light therapy
DNRS

Then, work on specifics using the info in the reference's sections of this book.

Remember there are waves, bumps, and a rollercoaster ride. When you mobilise the bad things; try to enjoy the ride. There will also be layers to deal with, so always reassess every three months.

You also don't have to do everything but start with something.

Don't be too hard on yourself!

Give yourself time to heal!

Do the questionnaires in the journal and on the website to assess your exposure to potential bad things. This is where you see you are exposed in a certain area, focus on reducing that exposure, then track your symptoms and notice the small changes in your symptoms, that eventually become big changes with time.

Chapter 26: Track and Reset Yourself.

Start by doing a "readiness to change assessment". In my experience, you can't force someone who is not willing to make changes, to make the changes they need to heal. They must be ready to put in the work and if they aren't ready then they need to undergo therapy to assess why or try a different approach that might work better for them until they are ready. The stages of change are:

- Pre-contemplation (Not yet acknowledging that there is a problem behaviour that needs to be changed), such as changing their diet, relationships, habits and more.
- Contemplation (Acknowledging that there is a problem but not yet ready, sure of wanting, or lacks confidence to make a change).
- Preparation/Determination (Getting ready to change).
- Action/Willpower (Changing behaviour).
- Maintenance (Maintaining the behaviour change).

People must be at Contemplation at the very least before they are able to do a full Reset!

The basics to cover would be - How ready are you to:

- Significantly modify your diet if needed
- Take nutritional supplements each day, if needed
- Journal what you eat and how you feel each day
- Modify your lifestyle - e.g., work demands
- Improve your sleep habits
- Practice a relaxation technique
- Engage in regular exercise
- Recognise toxic relationships

Ideally the answer should all be "Very willing," but if you notice that there are areas where you are less willing to change, then at least become aware of that block and work on that willingness!

The next step is to reduce exposure.

TOXIN EXPOSURE

G General Exposure **H** Heavy metals **P** Persistent Chemicals **M** Moulds **R** Relationships

	Question	YES OFTEN	YES SOMETIMES	IN THE PAST YEAR	NO NEVER
G	Do you eat highly processed foods (i.e., foods with added artificial colours, flavours, preservatives, or sweeteners), deep-fried, or fast foods?	3	2	1	0
G	Do you drink carbonated drinks, with or without sugar more than once a week?	3	2	1	0
G	Do you regularly consume more than 14 units of alcohol per week?	3	2	1	0
G	Do you live or work near a source of electromagnetic radiation (i.e., cell phone tower, high-voltage power lines, or other known source)?	3	2	1	0
G	Do you often travel by air, more than once a month?	3	2	1	0
G	Are you sensitive to smoke, perfumes, fragrances, cleaning products, gasoline, or other fumes?	3	2	1	0
G	Do you have any unusual reactions to anaesthesia or to prescription or over-the-counter medications?	3	2	1	0
G	Do you have food reactions, sensitivities, or intolerances that you are aware of?	3	2	1	0
G	Do you have environmental allergies?	3	2	1	0
H	Do you regularly eat canned or farmed fish and seafood?	3	2	1	0
H	Do you cook using aluminium or copper pans?	3	2	1	0
H	Are you aware of exposure to toxic substances (i.e., treated lumber, lead paint, paint chips or dust, broken mercury thermometers or fluorescent bulbs, etc.) at home or work?	3	2	1	0
H	Are you exposed to toxic chemicals as a result of a hobby (i.e., paints, photo-developing chemicals, epoxy adhesives, glues, varnishes, etc.)?	3	2	1	0
H	Do you have root canals, extracted teeth, "silver" fillings, crowns, dental sealants, dentures, retainers, aligning trays, braces, mouth guards, dental implants, etc.?	3	2	1	0
H	Do you have any artificial materials in your body (implants, pins, joints, etc.)?	3	2	1	0
H	Do you drink unfiltered water from a well, spring, or cistern, or from old plumbing pipes?	3	2	1	0
H	Do you live or work near an industrial pollution source (i.e., highway, factory, incinerator, gas station, power plant, etc.)?	3	2	1	0
H	Do you have wood-burning, propane, or gas stoves or appliances at home or work?	3	2	1	0
H	Do you smoke, or are you often exposed to second-hand smoke?	3	2	1	0
M	Do you regularly eat leftovers? (more than a day old)	3	2	1	0
M	Does your home or workplace show signs of mould or water damage (i.e., cracking paint, ceiling leaks, decaying insulation or foam, visible mould or the smell of mould, or damp windows, basement, or crawlspaces, etc.)?	3	2	1	0
M	Has your car had any obvious water damage or does it have a musty smell?	3	2	1	0
M	Do you live or work in a sealed building with recirculated air?	3	2	1	0
M	Do you live near a body of water?	3	2	1	0
P	Are conventional cleaning chemicals, disinfectants, hand sanitisers, air fresheners, scented candles, or other scented products used at your home or work?	3	2	1	0
P	Does your home or workplace contain new construction materials or furniture (i.e., paint, laminate flooring, particle board, new carpeting, bedding, furniture, etc.)?	3	2	1	0
P	Do you regularly eat conventionally-farmed (not certified organic) or genetically-modified fruits and vegetables?	3	2	1	0
P	Do you regularly eat conventionally/factory farmed animal products? (i.e., meat, poultry, dairy, eggs)	3	2	1	0
P	Do you store and/or reheat food in plastic containers?	3	2	1	0
P	Do you live or work in an agricultural area or another type of area where you are exposed to herbicides, pesticides, or fungicides?	3	2	1	0
P	Are you a regular golfer?	3	2	1	0
P	Do you use conventional beauty or personal care products?	3	2	1	0
R	Do you have any close relationships that are non supportive and potentially destructive?	3	2	1	0

G = /27 H = /30 M = /15 P = /24 R = /3

TOTAL = /99

30 day RESET program

I have had excellent success with my patients who are poor detoxifiers or have high toxic burden (or both). You can make this program more designed to you by doing a food sensitivity test and specifically removing any reactive foods and then reintroducing them later. Just a note on food sensitivity tests is that the markers assessed can be rehabilitated. This means you won't necessarily be sensitive to a food flagged as being sensitive, forever. You need to retest until you have no more sensitivities. The sensitivities are an indicator that you are not chewing, digesting and absorbing your food correctly so you will need to work on gut health to improve the food sensitivities!

Food sensitivity testing isn't essential, but I have seen some good results when a test is used. There are a few on the market, so if you want to get tested, maybe speak to someone who works in nutrition for advice.

The program is also best done using a medical food supplement along with an omega 3 and a probiotic, but if you don't want to use these then please opt for the best quality food you can get. Medical foods are not protein shakes! They are meals designed with a function so you can get one for detoxification generally, for liver or kidney support, for gut health, sugar balance or even inflammation! Use one or more to get the best results. If you cannot source a medical food, then a good quality protein shake, and liver support supplement can be used.

How you determine what you can eat

Eat like your ancestors! If they wouldn't recognise the food on your plate, then chances are you would be better off eating something else.

Chose fresh, local, organic and regenerative where possible. I have separated the categories of foods into sections based on whether you can eat liberally or should rather avoid:

Eat liberally:

You can enjoy as much of these foods as you like. No counting calories or calculating ratios of protein, fat or carbohydrate. This isn't a "cleanse" or a fast. If a food is on this list, you're free to eat it.

Organ meats (especially liver): Liver is the most nutrient-dense food on the planet. If you don't like the taste of liver, one good trick is to put one chicken liver in each cube of an ice cube tray and freeze them. Then, when you're making any meat dish, dice up one chicken liver and add it to the meat. Pate is also a good way to get your daily dose of liver.

Bone broth soups: It's essential to balance your intake of muscle meats and organ meats with homemade bone broths. Bone broths are rich in glycine, and amino acid found in collagen, which is a protein important in maintaining a healthy gut lining.

Fish: Especially fatty fish, like salmon, mackerel and herring. Wild is preferable. You need to eat three 6 oz or 170gm servings of fatty fish per week to balance your omega-6 to omega-3 ratio.

Vegetables: All non-starchy vegetables are considered core vegetables. Choose different colours and different sources of those colours each week, use the charts to select for the week. Cooked and raw. When you are asked to only eat core vegetables, limit the starchy vegetables like yams, sweet potatoes, yucca/manioc, taro, lotus root, etc. on the days indicated. Specifically, days 8-17.

Fermented vegetables and fruits. (unless you are mouldy) Sauerkraut, kimchi, kefir, etc. These are excellent for gut health. If you are mould toxic, stick to Kefir and leave the rest. If you have histamine sensitivity (get red and itchy easily) then avoid all the fermented foods.

Traditional fats. Butter and olive oil, olives, avocados and coconuts (including coconut milk). Are all allowed throughout

Earth and sea salt and all spices. Eat with each meal where possible as they have loads of healing ingredients.

Beverages: Filtered water. Herbal teas

Eat in moderation:

You can eat these foods, but don't go wild with them. In general, you want to limit consumption of these foods compared to those in the "eat liberally" category.

Meat and poultry: Unless specified to avoid, as on days 8-17, or you choose to avoid them, you can eat them Emphasise grass fed meats like beef and lamb, but also free-range pork, chicken, turkey, duck and wild game like venison, ostrich, etc. Organic and free-range is always preferable but is especially so during this program.

Eggs. Preferably free-range and organic. Avoid on days 8-17.

Whole fruit: Approximately 1-3 servings per day, depending on your blood sugar balance. Favour low sugar fruits like apples & pears, berries and peaches over tropical fruits. On days 8-17 you should only eat apples and pears. Then reintroduce berries as per the chart.

Nuts and seeds: A maximum of a handful per day are allowed at the beginning and end of the program. Preferably soaked overnight and dehydrated or roasted at low temperature (150 degrees) to improve digestibility. Favour nuts lower in omega-6, like hazelnuts and macadamias, and minimise nuts high in omega-6, like brazil nuts and almonds. Avoid totally if you are mould toxic.

Legumes: Green beans, sugar peas and snap peas. Beans of all kinds (soy, black, kidney, pinto, etc.), peas, lentils are allowed except for days 8-17, unless you are vegetarian, then you can eat them throughout.

Dark chocolate. 70% or higher in small amounts is permitted.

Dairy. Including butter, cheese, yogurt, milk, cream & any dairy product that comes from a cow, goat or sheep. Avoid if you suspect an intolerance and on days 7-17.

Grains. Including sourdough bread, rice, cereal, oats, or any gluten-free pseudo grains like sorghum, teff, quinoa, amaranth, buckwheat, are all allowed as per the schedule. On days 8-17 you will only be allowed quinoa and rice.

Locally source honey.

Avoid completely:

Yep, completely. This is where the rubber hits the road. The success (or failure) of the program hinges on your ability to steer clear of these foods during the 30-day Reset.

Try to eat as much variety as possible, don't get trapped into eating the same thing for breakfast. Lunch and dinner... in fact, eat something totally different for each meal each day!

Gluten: Wheat, Barley rye etc.

Restaurant food. The main problem with eating out is that restaurants cook with industrial seed oils, which wreak havoc on the body and cause serious inflammation. You don't need to become a cave dweller, but it's best to limit eating out as much as possible during this initial period.

Concentrated sweeteners, real or artificial. Including sugar, high fructose corn syrup, maple syrup, agave, brown rice syrup, Splenda, Equal, NutraSweet, xylitol, stevia, etc.

Processed or refined foods. As a rule, if it comes in a bag or a box, don't eat it. This also includes highly processed "health foods" like energy bars, dairy-free creamers, etc.

Industrial seed oils. Soybean, corn, safflower, sunflower, cottonseed, canola, etc. Read labels - seed oils are in almost all processed, packaged and refined foods (which you should be mostly avoiding anyway).

Drinks: Sodas and diet sodas. All forms. Alcohol. In any form. (Don't freak out. It's just 30 days.) And coffee on certain parts of the program.

Processed sauces and seasonings. Soy sauce, tamari, and other processed seasonings and sauces (which often have sugar, soy, gluten, or all of the above).

The stages of the program

This program is a 4 step, 30-day, modified elimination diet with loads of nutritional support! I also advise that you sauna, get mild movement and ensure healthy sleep and stress management while on the program.

The Reset program is designed to reduce inflammation, improve digestion, burn fat, identify food sensitivities, reduce allergic reactions, boost energy, regulate blood sugar and stabilise mood.

After completing the Reset you'll have a bit more leeway to go off the rails every now and then. After all, there's more to life than healthy food and chewing food!

By removing the foods that most commonly cause problems, you allow your body to reset and recover from whatever symptoms those foods have been provoking. Just one cheat could trigger a whole new cascade of reactions. Don't do it. It's not worth it.

Remember, 30 days is just a minimum. Some people may need 45, 60 or even 90 days to get the full benefits of the Reset program, but some see amazing results in just 2 weeks, so you do you and repeat the process as often as you need to!

Step 1 - preparation days 1 & 2

During this stage, you will plan your coming week, get rid of any temptations in your kitchen and home, start buying the first weeks' worth of groceries. Start your journal, noting why you are doing the program and how you are feeling. You will start your daily broth and focus on chewing. Get a 30 second hourglass and chew until all the sand has drained, then you can take your next bite and repeat.

Step 2 - Initial Clearing —Days 3-7:

Begin to eliminate potentially allergenic foods as summarised in the Daily Schedule Chart below, or in the journal, while you slowly increase intake of allowed foods and introduce the nutritional supplements. The aim is to support the body by building up its supply of protein and plant bioflavonoids, while also working on stress & sleep and ensuring healthy gut function.

Step 3 - Metabolic Detoxification— Days 8-14:

You will be eating from a limited menu and increasing foods that support detoxification as well as supplements as indicated or recommended by your healthcare provider. This is generally considered the hardest week due to the strict restrictions and some people experience mild to moderate detox symptoms, such as headache, joint pain, changes in bowel movements. These are often symptoms they have experienced in the past and some people get nervous about getting worse, but it is simply a layer of toxins being mobilised and removed from the body.

Metabolic Detoxification— Days 15-17:

Remove sweeteners completely. You're almost past the worst of it, look forward to the next stage! This is generally where people see some improvement in brain fog, joint pain and sleep.

Step 4 - Days 18 & 19: Reintroduction begins.

Reintroduce eggs, non-gluten grains and starches, as well as dairy. Legumes and berries starchy seasonal vegetables can also be reintroduced. Please track how your body reacts to the food that is being reintroduced.

Day 20: Almost there!

Add grass fed meat, nuts and seeds as well as locally sourced honey.

Days 21-29: The home stretch

Well done! You can now add back all fruits protein from all sources as well as the allowed sweeteners

Day 30 & Beyond: Maintenance

You're finished and you can celebrate with some mould free coffee or a small glass of organic wine!

Continue with your daily essentials (the food and supplements that support your genetic susceptibilities) for ongoing nutritional support for detoxification to keep you feeling better long term.

The companion journal is designed to help you through the 30 days. It has the questionnaires and daily journaling with motivation along the way. There is room to do the program twice so you can repeat it if you need to. You can scan the QR code to go directly to the site.

Caveats and tweaks

With certain health conditions the basic program above needs further modification.

Those with arthritis, joint pain, autoimmune disease and severe gut issues should also eliminate nightshades and eggs.

Nightshades include:

- Potatoes
- Tomatoes

- Sweet and hot peppers
- Eggplant
- tomatillos, pepinos, pimentos, paprika and cayenne pepper.

Nightshades have compounds called alkaloids that can cause inflammation and worsen joint pain in susceptible people. Eggs contain proteins that are common allergens, particularly in susceptible people. Kale and spinach can also be a problem for some inflamed people especially if they are eaten raw and in large quantities.

Those with insulin resistance, hypoglycaemia or reactive hypoglycaemia, and those wishing to lose weight, should limit fruit and starchy vegetables. The total amount eaten each day should equal roughly 50 grams per day of carbohydrate, which is the amount contained in 2 servings of low-glycaemic fruit (berries) and 1-2 servings of starch (i.e. sweet potato, taro, yucca, etc.).

Those with fatigue, insomnia, anxiety, mood swings or depression should eliminate coffee, tea, green tea and all caffeine entirely. Caffeine stimulates the adrenals and can worsen all these conditions. Once your adrenal issues have been addressed, you may be able to add them back in moderation.

Recommended supplements to source are:

- Medical food
- Omega 3 from a reliable brand
- A probiotic
- A liver support formula
- Stay on anything else recommended by your Healthcare provider

Enjoy the process!

The next few pages have some tools and guide you can use. These are also found in the companion journal and the website http://www.drshania.com/.

DAILY SCHEDULE

	Days 1-2	Days 3-7	Days 8-14	Days 15-17	Days 18-19	Day 20	Days 21-29	Days 30+
Bone broth	1 cup	1 cup	1-2 cup	1-2 cup	1-2 cup	1 cup	1 cup	1 cup
Fruits	✓	✓	Apples and pears only	Apples and pears only	Apples, berries and pears only	All seasonal fruit only	✓	✓
Vegetables	✓	✓	Non-startchy, seasonal veg only	Non-startchy, seasonal veg only	All seasonal veg only	All seasonal veg only	✓	✓
Animal proteins	✓	All regenerative and wild meats, including liver and organs.	Fish and liver only	Fish and liver only	Fish and liver only	Fish, liver and grass fed meats only	Fish and grass fed meats and liver or organ meats only	✓
Eggs	✓	✓	✓	✗	✓	✓	✓	✓
Plant based proteins	✓	Beans, legumes (lentils &peas), Hummus	✗	✗	Beans, legumes (lentils &peas), Hummus	Beans, legumes (lentils &peas), Hummus	✓	✓
Beverages	✓	Green tea, herbal teas, water - unlimited	Green tea, herbal teas, water - unlimited	Green tea, herbal teas, water - unlimited	Green tea, herbal teas, water - unlimited	Green tea, herbal teas, water - unlimited	Green tea, herbal teas, water - unlimited	✓
Fresh or dried herbs & spices	✓	✓	✓	✓	✓	✓	✓	✓
Oils & fats	✓	Avocado, butter, coconut, flax, grapeseed, olive and sesame oils	Avocado, butter, coconut, flax, grapeseed, olive and sesame oils	Avocado, butter, coconut, flax, grapeseed, olive and sesame oils	Avocado, butter, coconut, flax, grapeseed, olive and sesame oils	Avocado, butter, coconut, flax, grapeseed, olive and sesame oils	Avocado, butter, coconut, flax, grapeseed, olive and sesame oils	✓
Grains and starches	✓	Gluten free grains and starches	Quinoa and whole rice only	Quinoa and whole rice only	Gluten free grains and starches	Gluten free grains and starches	Gluten free grains and starches	✓
Dairy	✓	✓	Dairy alternatives example: coconut milk	Dairy alternatives example: coconut milk	Whole milk and cheese	Whole milk and cheese	✓	✓
Whole nuts and seeds	✓	✓	✗	✗	✗	✓	✓	✓
Natural sweeteners	✓		Locally sourced honey	✗	✗	Locally sourced honey	✓	✓
Medical food (protein shake)	Not needed	1-2 Scoops as needed 1-2 times a day	2 Scoops 3 times a day as needed	2 Scoops 3 times a day as needed	2 Scoops 3 times a day as needed	2 Scoops 3 times a day as needed	1-2 Scoops as needed 1-2 times a day	If you feel you need it you can continue

* Vegetarians can skip this and maintain their plant based protein intake

✗ None allowed   ✓ Any allowed

You can download the colourful high resolution images off 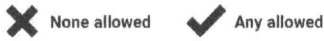www.drshania.com.

RED FOODS

Beans (adzuki, kidney, red), Beetroot, Red peppers, Blood oranges, Cranberries, Cherries, Goji berries, Grapefruit (pink), Red apples, Red grapes, Red onions, Red plums, Pomegranate, Potatoes (red skin), Radicchio, Red cabbage, Red leaf lettuce, Radishes, Raspberries, Strawberries, Sweet red peppers, Rhubarb, Rooibos tea, Tomato, Watermelon.

BENEFITS

Cancer protective, healthy inflammatory response, cell protection, gastrointestinal health, heart health, hormone balance, liver health.

YELLOW FOODS

Apple, Banana, Bell peppers (yellow), Sweetcorn, Corn-on-the-cob, Chickpeas, Ginger root, Lemon, Millet, Pineapple, Popcorn.

BENEFITS

Cancer protective, immune health, cell protection, Cancer protective, healthy inflammatory response cell protection, cognition, skin health, eye health, heart/vascular health.

BLUE/PURPLE/BLACK FOODS

Aubergine, Berries (blue/black), Cabbage (purple), Carrots (purple), Cauliflower (purple), Figs, Grapes (purple), Kale (purple), Olives (black), Plums, Potatoes (purple), Prunes, Raisins, Rice (black/purple).

BENEFITS

Cancer protective, healthy inflammatory response cell protection, cognition health, heart health, liver

ORANGE FOODS

Apricots, Bell peppers (orange), Carrots, Grapefruit, Mango, Nectarine, Orange, Papaya, Pumpkin, Squash (Butternut/Acorn/Winter), Sweet Potato, Tangerines, Turmeric Root, Yams.

BENEFITS

Cancer protective, immune health, cell protection, reduced all-cause mortality, immune health, reproductive health, skin health, source of pro-vitamin A.

GREEN FOODS

Apples (green), Artichoke, Asparagus, Avocado, Bamboo shoots, Bean sprouts, Bok Choy, Broccoli, Brussels sprouts, Cabbage (Beet leaves, chard, dandelion leaves, kale, lettuce, mustard leaves, spinach, rocket, etc), Celery, Cucumbers, Edemame (soyabeans), Beans, Peas (e.g. green, mangetout), Green tea, Lettuce, Limes, Okra, Olives (green), Rosemary, Spinach, Watercress.

BENEFITS

Healthy inflammatory response, brain health, cell protection, skin health, hormone balance, heart health, liver health.a

WHITE/TAN/BROWN FOODS

Apples, Beans (butter, cannellini, etc), Cauliflower, Cinnamon, Clove, Coconut, Cocoa, Coffee, Dark Chocolate, Flaxseed, Garlic, Ginger, Hummus, Legumes (chickpeas, dried beans, Hummus, Houmous, Lentils, Peanuts, etc), Mushrooms, Nuts (almonds, cashews, macadamias, pecans, walnuts), Onions, Pears, Seeds (flax, hemp, pumpkin, seasame, sunflower, etc), Shallots, Tahini, Tea (black, white), Whole grains (amaranth, buckwheat, corn, millet, montina, oats, quinoa, rice, sorghum, teff - all naturally free of gluten).

BENEFITS

Cancer protective, anti-microbial, cell protection, gastrointestinal health, heart health, liver health, hormone balance.

Chapter 27 – Reference Section for Toxic and Essential Elements

Aluminium (Al)

The nature of aluminium

Hot & Dry – Aluminium will suck the wet out of anything! It is used in anti-perspirants for this very reason. When you have lots of Aluminium in you, expect dry skin or eczema and psoriasis as well as colic or constipation and issues with memory as it dries up the brain (Aluminium is linked to Alzheimer's).

Role in the body

Aluminium is a unique element as it has no supported uses in nature, not one. Aluminium is neither required by biological systems nor is it known to participate in any essential biological processes. While today all living organisms contain possess some a certain amount of aluminium within them. However, there is no scientific evidence that any organism uses it for any biological purpose. As it is such a useful; metal in our day-to-day lives, there is a high likelihood of a positive aluminium result in a hair, urine, or blood test as it is so prevalent in daily life.

Before the industrial revolution, Aluminium was a metal that was tightly bound into the earth until we found that it has so many uses. Now it is mined wherever it is found and used in a huge vast variety of products, including cans, foils, kitchen utensils, window frames, beer kegs, and aeroplane parts. This is because of its properties, such as the fact that it is extremely incredibly light weight, corrosion resistant, is an excellent heat and electricity conductor, and, in relation to its weight, is almost twice as good a conductor as copper.

The metal itself is also considered by the industry to be non-toxic and odourless, which makes it ideal for packaging sensitive products such as food or pharmaceuticals. As for its toxicity, if it is heated (such as cooking) or exposed to acids, aluminium will leach into the food that it is exposed to. This accumulation of the metal can create a burden that impacts health.

Sources of aluminium

After oxygen and silicon, aluminium is the most abundant element in the crust of the earth.

Aluminium is used to produce beverage cans, cooking pots, aluminium foil and cooking with these can expose you to it. Exposure from food cooked in aluminium cookware is made worse when the food is acidic. Fluoridated water increases the leaching of aluminium from aluminium pots and pans.

Exposure to aluminium is ubiquitous via food, water, air and soil but in particular:

- Aluminium foil and old cooking
- Anti-perspirants
- Buffered aspirin
- Cannabis smoke
- Congenital – from mom to her baby
- Aluminium containing antacids
- Drinking water (aluminium is frequently added to municipal water during flocculation)
- Some dental amalgams
- Baking powders
- Drying agents in salt and other food additive products
- Processed cheese
- Bleached flour
- Dialysis

There are more sources as it is so extensively used in industry, but these are the main ones.

How to assess body burden

Whole blood, serum, hair, urine can all be used to assess aluminium exposure.

The best way to assess aluminium burden is through hair tissue mineral analysis.

Blood would only pick up a recent exposure.

Urine pre and post-challenge tests will also reveal excess aluminium. Urine may show a rise in a post Calcium disodium ethylene diamine tetra acetic acid (EDTA) dose. This chelator has been found to be effective in removing aluminium from patients affected by neurological disorders. Malic acid has also been found to be effective in increasing the urinary excretion of aluminium, and citric acids are said to be effective in increasing improving the faecal excretion of aluminium.

Total porphyrin elevation can also be measured in a urine test via specialised labs.

How aluminium affects health

The major tissue sites of aluminium toxicity are the nervous system, digestive system, immune system, bone, liver, and red blood cells, and aluminium may interfere with haem (porphyrin) synthesis.

Nervous System - Aluminium can negatively impact the nervous system in humans. It can affect neurotransmission by blocking the formation of calcium-permeable ion channels, which can inhibit the increase in calcium influx induced by neurotrophic factors such as the brain-derived neurotrophic factor. This may be why it leads to decrease in memory and the associated neurodegenerative diseases like dementia and Alzheimer's. The presence of aluminium in the brain can contribute to any ongoing degenerative conditions such as Alzheimer's disease or multiple sclerosis, ultimately resulting in earlier onset and/or more aggressive forms of the disease. Aluminium also induces neuronal apoptosis. In other words, nerve cells commit suicide in the presence of Aluminium.

Digestive System - Aluminium reduces intestinal activity, and, by doing so, can cause colic. Aluminium intake may negatively affect intestinal microbiota.

Bones: Aluminium replaces calcium in bone, disrupting normal osteoid formation and mineralization. Aluminium interrupts calcium exchange, preventing renal resorption of calcium. Aluminium effectively interferes with the normal physiologic control of parathyroid hormone, and therefore may impact the conversion of vitamin D to its active form.

Red blood cells (RBC): Administration of aluminium alone produces increased free erythrocyte proto-porphyrins and decreased iron concentrations in RBC, spleen and blood.

Toxicity symptoms

Abnormal speech, myoclonic jerks, osteomalacia, progressive encephalopathy, Alzheimer's disease, Parkinson's disease

Early symptoms of aluminium burden or toxicity include

Alzheimer's disease or dementia   Heartburn and an aversion to meat

Amyotrophic lateral sclerosis

Anaemia

Burning pain in head relieved by food

Colic or flatulence

Dental cavities

Dryness of skin and mucosa

Headaches

Hypoparathyroidism

Kidney dysfunction

Liver dysfunction

Neuromuscular disorders

Osteomalacia

Parkinson's disease

Peptic ulcer

Protective measures

Assessing copper, zinc and iron status helps to determine a patient's vulnerability to the toxic effects of aluminium, and appropriate elemental treatments may help to overcome aluminium toxicity.

Iron - Iron deficiency predisposes to higher aluminium absorption and, conversely, aluminium decreases absorption and uptake of iron.

Magnesium - The toxic effect of aluminium was less marked when magnesium was present at a higher concentration (antagonistic inhibition). The best form would be Magnesium malate.

B Vitamins, Zinc, Vitamin C, and Vitamin E will all help to reduce the toxic effects of aluminium.

Other nutrient therapies which that improve the activity of the liver, kidneys, bowel, and the skin can be helpful!

A healthy, organic diet high in green and colourful vegetables, grass-fed red meat, nuts, and whole grains is also important essential as is they include the following:

- Cilantro/coriander
- Garlic
- Blueberries
- Cold-pressed unrefined organic coconut oil
- Chia and flaxseed
- Milk thistle
- Vitamin C (and foods rich in this vitamin)

- Spirulina and chlorella
- Fresh, filtered water (and plenty of it!)

Specific binders

Silica has been found to reduce aluminium levels drastically in the body. It does this by binding with its molecules and extracting them out of brain cells and ultimately out of the body through urine and other means.

Deferoxamine, also known as desferrioxamine and sold under the brand name Desferal, is a medication that binds iron and aluminium. It is specifically used in iron overdose, haemochromatosis either due to multiple blood transfusions or an underlying genetic condition, and aluminium toxicity in people on dialysis.

What does detoxing feel like

Detoxing aluminium will exaggerate the associated symptoms, such as dryness, for a few days as it moves from storage. Fatigue and constipation are common as are flare ups in dry skin conditions.

Further testing

Further testing of an aluminium-toxic patient might involve measurement of bone resorption, urinary catecholamines, oxidative stress, and even vitamin D.

Antimony (Sb)

Nature of antimony

Antimony has no specific nature, however; it interferes with glutathione and increases oxidative stress.

Role in the body

Antimony is a potentially toxic element with no known biological function. Although it is less toxic than arsenic, antimony is a similar group V metalloid with the capacity to interrupt enzyme sulfhydryl groups.

Sources of antimony

Antimony and its compounds have been used in various industrial applications, such as flame retardants, alloys, and semiconductors.

Antimony is present in cosmetic products. Please check your products.

Other materials containing antimony include alloys, ceramics, glass, plastic and synthetic fabrics.

Antimony is present in incinerators, smelters and fossil- fuel combustion, thus can be in contaminated air.

How to assess body burden

Because whole-blood antimony is cleared from the blood slowly over months, it best reflects chronic exposure.

Urine has shown good correlation with acute antimony exposure.

Hair analysis can also be used in cases of chronic exposure.

How antimony affects health

Respiratory Effects: Inhalation of antimony dust or fumes can irritate the respiratory system, leading to symptoms such as coughing, difficulty breathing, wheezing, and chest tightness. Prolonged exposure to high levels of antimony in occupational settings may contribute to chronic respiratory conditions.

Skin and Eye Irritation: Direct contact with antimony or its compounds can cause skin and eye irritation. It may lead to redness, itching, rash, and discomfort. Eye exposure can result in conjunctivitis or corneal damage.

Gastrointestinal Effects: Ingestion of large amounts of antimony or its compounds can irritate the gastrointestinal tract. Symptoms may include nausea, vomiting, abdominal pain, diarrhoea, and gastrointestinal inflammation.

Cardiovascular Effects: Some studies suggest that chronic exposure to antimony may affect the cardiovascular system. It may lead to changes in blood pressure, heart rate, and electrocardiogram (ECG) abnormalities. However, the exact precise mechanisms and clinical significance of these effects are still being under investigation.

Kidney and Liver Damage: Prolonged exposure to high levels of antimony can potentially damage the kidneys and liver. It may lead to kidney dysfunction, liver inflammation, and cellular damage in these organs.

It's worth noting that the toxicity of antimony depends on the specific form and concentration of exposure, as well as the duration and route of exposure. Occupational settings, such as antimony mining, refining, or manufacturing industries, pose a higher risk of exposure. Environmental contamination or consumption of contaminated food or water sources may also contribute to exposure.

Toxicity symptoms

Antimony toxicity presents with nausea, vomiting, abdominal pain, haematuria (blood in the urine), haemolytic anaemia and renal failure. Subclinical exposure could result in increased reactive oxygen species and increased apoptosis.

Protective measures

Antimony is excreted via bile and urine as a glutathione conjugate, so supporting glutathione is key. Symptomatic treatment and possibly chelation therapy would be needed in acute exposure, for chronic low-grade exposure, remove the source, ensure good gut health, and support phase 2 detoxification.

To mitigate the risks associated with antimony exposure, occupational safety measures, and proper handling protocols should be followed in industrial settings. Additionally, adherence to regulatory guidelines and standards for antimony use and disposal can help minimise environmental contamination.

If you have concerns about antimony exposure or suspect exposure-related symptoms, it is recommended to consult with a healthcare professional or poison control centre for appropriate evaluation, guidance, and treatment.

Specific binders

N-Acetyl cysteine and DMSA.

What does detoxing feel like

No specific sensations are known

Further testing

Assessing glutathione and overall oxidative stress would be useful.

Arsenic (As)

The nature of arsenic

Arsenic affects almost every system in the body. Its nature is to produce burning pains, and in an acute exposure, it specifically affects explicitly the guts and can cause symptoms that are often confused for food poisoning, where there is burning pain and often diarrhoea, if the exposure is chronic, it may even be excreted through the skin producing a psoriasis-like lesion with a white powdery look. It can also be identified by characteristic horizontal white lines across the finger and toenails, these are call Mee's lines.

Role in the body

Arsenic affects multiple enzymes and organ systems and is deadly at high enough doses. Arsenic is infamous for its use in homicide by poisoning, exists in toxic and non-toxic forms. The toxic forms are the inorganic species of arsenic, As-III and As-V. Preserved "pressure-treated" wood contains appreciable amounts of the toxic forms of arsenic, as do many insecticides. The organoarsines, arsenobetaine and arsenocholine are non-toxic forms of arsenic that are present in many foods, especially shellfish and other predators such as cod and haddock in the seafood chain. This is why we ask people to refrain from eat these fish before doing a urine test, as they may have a false positive of harmless arsenic in their urine results.

Arsenic has long held a position of ambiguity regarding its activity in biological systems. Despite the recognised toxicity of many forms of arsenic, various arsenicals have been used in the practice of medicine. A specific nutritional role for inorganic arsenic has been uncovered only recently, but animal feeds have been supplemented with "growth-promoting" organic arsenical additives for many years. Another curious feature of arsenic biochemistry is the ability of the element partially to counteract the ill effects of yet another potentially toxic substance, selenium.

Arsenic expresses its toxicity by:

- Binding with sulfhydryl groups, which causes distortion of protein structure and loss of enzyme activity.
- Tightly binding dihydrolipoic acid, a necessary cofactor for keto acid dehydrogenases.

- Competing with phosphate for binding to ATP during its mitochondrial synthesis, decreasing phosphorylation of ADP, thus affecting energy.

Sources of arsenic

The most common sources are metal foundry, drinking water, seafood, glues, industrial exposure, contaminated wine, contaminated herbal supplements, cigarette smoke, arsenic-treated wood (often found in playgrounds) and of course poisoning. Rice and seafood are also a common source of exposure.

Arsenic is the 20th most abundant element on earth. The inorganic forms, such as arsenite and arsenate compounds, are lethal to humans and other organisms in the environment and are not commonly found. However, less immediately toxic forms are more prevalent. Humans get in contact with to arsenic occurs through several various means, which includes industrial sources such as smelting and microelectronic industries.

Drinking water may be contaminated with arsenic, which is present in wood preservatives, herbicides, pesticides, fungicides, and paints. Organic arsenic (arsenate) is found in a variety of various foods such as chicken, fish, shellfish, and rice, so please reduce those if your levels are high, but remember that this is the less toxic form. Fish, shellfish, meat, poultry, dairy products, rice and cereals can also be dietary sources of arsenic, although exposure from these foods is generally much lower compared to exposure through contaminated groundwater. In seafood, arsenic is mainly found in its less toxic organic form.

Rice is known to accumulate around ten times as much arsenic as other cereals. In rice grains arsenic is concentrated in the outer bran layer surrounding the endosperm. This means that brown rice, (un-milled or unpolished rice that retains its bran) contains more arsenic than white rice.

Inorganic arsenate or arsenite is more environmental and much more toxic and can be from contaminated water, pesticides, tobacco, beer, table salt, paint, cosmetics, pigments, rat poison, glass and mirror manufacture, fungicides, and wood preservatives.

How to assess body burden

Whole blood is suitable for identifying acute exposure to arsenic, and high levels should be addressed immediately.

Urinary arsenic is most measured to screen for arsenic exposure because levels reflect intake from all sources. Urine reflects arsenic exposure in the few days prior to specimen collection. Urinary inorganic (toxic) arsenic peaks at about 10 hours and returns to normal 20 to 30 hours after ingestion. Non- toxic organic arsenic is completely excreted in 24 to 48 hours after ingestion. Patients should abstain from eating seafood for 48 hours prior to testing because of the high content of non-toxic organoarsines in most seafood.

Because most arsenic leaves your body within a few hours of exposure, analysis of your blood or urine cannot detect if you were exposed to arsenic more than 12-30 hours ago.

Arsenite accumulates in the hair tissue as it has a strong affinity to bind to keratin, so hair analysis is considered a valuable means of detecting past arsenic exposure and toxicity.

How arsenic affects health

Arsenic is a potent enzyme inhibitor and affects all systems! As it also interferes with ATP it affects anything that your body needs energy for!

Arsenic also interferes with uptake of folic acid, thus affecting methylation.

With the inhibition of sulfhydryl enzyme systems such as Glutathione, there is increased oxidative stress to all systems. Glutathione contains a sulfhydryl group and is involved in many cellular processes, including the detoxification of xenobiotics and the regulation of protein function

Toxicity symptoms

Lethal arsenic poisoning is characterised by toxic hepatitis and pancreatitis, neurological dysfunction, respiratory difficulty, renal failure and cardiovascular disturbance. Exposure to arsenic-laden drinking water can induce symptoms of gastroenteritis and lead to cancer, diabetes, and neurological and vascular dysfunction. Arsenic can cause skin cancer and dermatosis.

Symptoms of acute arsenic toxicity include pain, eye irritation, nausea, vomiting, and diarrhoea, characteristic skin lesions, decreased production of red and white blood cells, abnormal heart function, blood vessel damage, liver and/or kidney damage, and impaired nerve function causing a "pins-and-needles" feeling. In cases of extreme exposure, arsenic is fatal, with a lethal dose being as little as one to 25 mg arsenic per kg of body weight.

Other symptoms can include any of the following:

Abdominal pain and diarrhoea	Kidney damage
Anorexia (loss of appetite)	Liver dysfunction and possibly jaundice
Dermatitis (with white powdery appearance - keratosis)	Muscle spasm and/or weakness
Diabetes	Pallor (grey appearance to the skin)
Fever	Peripheral neuritis
Hair loss	Oedema
Herpes flare ups (any version)	Vitiligo
Hypertension and abnormal ECG	Vertigo
Impaired healing	

Protective lifestyle measures

Identify the source and decrease the load where possible.

Cook rice using the method shown.

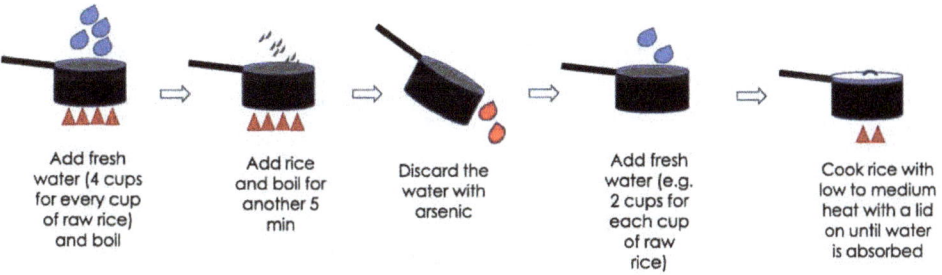

Add fresh water (4 cups for every cup of raw rice) and boil → Add rice and boil for another 5 min → Discard the water with arsenic → Add fresh water (e.g. 2 cups for each cup of raw rice) → Cook rice with low to medium heat with a lid on until water is absorbed

In all cases, selenium, Indian gooseberry, sulphur amino acids and glutathione can help protect against any damage being caused.

Arsenic needs to be methylated to be excreted, so supporting methylation is key to detoxification.

B vitamins, magnesium, and folate-rich foods such as liver, leafy greens, beets, asparagus, avocado, broccoli, to name a few.

Sulphur-rich foods and glutathione promotors are also useful.

Citrus pectin and Zeolite both bind to Arsenic in the gut and will help Phase 3 detoxification

Protective nutritional measures:

- Folate
- Iodine
- Selenium
- Sulphur
- Zinc
- Vitamin E
- Vitamin A

Specific binders

DMSA, DMPS, DMPA

Sacchyromyces proboulardi

N-Acetyl cysteine

Arsenicum Album as a homeopathic remedy in a low potency can also help.

What does detoxing feel like

When mobilising arsenic, there is often a flare up of the acute symptoms such as skin irritation and diarrhoea. As arsenic is very quickly metabolised, these symptoms should be short lived.

Further testing

Further testing would depend on the dose and duration of exposure. Assessing for diabetes and mitochondrial and microbial health would most likely be necessary.

Barium (Ba)

The nature of Barium

There is no real personality to barium. While barium itself is not highly toxic, certain forms of barium compounds can have adverse effects on the body when ingested, inhaled, or exposed to the skin.

Role in the body

Barium has no specific role in the body

Sources of barium

Barite is the primary commercial source of barium. It is a mineral composed mainly of barium sulphate ($BaSO_4$). Barite deposits can be found worldwide and are mined for industrial uses, including oil and gas drilling, paint manufacturing, and medical diagnostics.

Drinking Water: Barium can be present in drinking water sources, primarily due to natural leaching from geological formations or industrial contamination. The levels of barium in drinking water vary depending on the location and water source.

Food: Barium is naturally present in trace amounts in various foods. It can be found in fruits, vegetables, grains, seafood, and animal products. The levels of barium in food are generally low and considered safe for consumption.

Industrial Processes: Barium compounds, such as barium carbonate and barium chloride, are used in various industries, including glass manufacturing, ceramics, electronics, and paper production. These industrial processes can release barium into the environment.

Pharmaceuticals and Medical Uses: Barium compounds, particularly barium sulphate, are used in medical diagnostics as contrast agents for X-ray imaging. They are administered orally or rectally to enhance the visibility of certain specific organs and structures during imaging tests such as barium swallow or barium enema.

How to assess body burden

Urine and hair.

In a hair analysis, if you see a pattern of elevated calcium, magnesium, barium and strontium, indicates negative calcium balance. The paradoxical elevation of hair calcium in response to negative calcium balance apparently is a response of the hair follicular cells to elevated parathyroid hormone. The other three elements that typically become elevated, share with calcium the physiological responses to parathyroid hormone. Relatively small amounts of the elements mobilised from bone are passed into the highly metabolically active follicular cells, where they become sequestered in the extruded hair shaft. However, the high capacity of hair for divalent element binding can causes strong elevation of the concentrations in hair.

It's important to note that the toxicity of barium compounds can vary depending on the specific form, concentration, duration, and route of exposure. Occupational settings with high levels of barium exposure carry a higher risk. Additionally, proper handling and following safety guidelines in industries that use or produce barium are crucial to minimise exposure risks.

If you suspect barium exposure or experience symptoms related to barium toxicity, it is important crucial to seek medical attention promptly. Healthcare professionals can evaluate your symptoms, provide appropriate treatment, and offer guidance based on your specific circumstances.

How barium affects health

Gastrointestinal Effects: Barium compounds are commonly used as contrast agents in medical imaging tests, such as barium swallow or barium enema. When consumed orally, barium sulphate can temporarily coat the digestive system, allowing for better visualisation during X-rays. However, the ingestion of substantial large amounts of barium compounds or the use of inappropriate forms of barium can lead to gastrointestinal issues, including abdominal pain, nausea, vomiting, diarrhoea, and constipation.

Cardiovascular and Respiratory Effects: Inhalation or excessive exposure to certain forms of barium compounds, such as barium carbonate or barium chloride, can affect the cardiovascular and respiratory systems. These effects may include changes in heart rhythm (arrhythmias), increased blood pressure, difficulty breathing, and respiratory irritation.

Kidney and Liver Damage: Prolonged exposure to high levels of barium can potentially cause damage to the kidneys and liver. It may lead to kidney dysfunction, liver inflammation, and cellular damage in these organs.

Muscle Weakness: Barium compounds can interfere with the release of neurotransmitters in nerve-muscle junctions, which can result in muscle weakness and affect muscle function.

Baritosis: Prolonged occupational exposure to barium dust or aerosols can lead to a condition known as baritosis. It is characterised by the accumulation of barium particles in lung tissues, resulting in lung irritation, coughing, and respiratory symptoms.

Toxicity symptoms

These are rare but can include abdominal pain, nausea, vomiting, diarrhoea, and constipation, changes in heart rhythm (arrhythmias), increased blood pressure, difficulty breathing, and respiratory irritation.

Protective measures

Avoid exposure where possible and support phase 2 detoxification when exposed.

Specific binders

No specific binders

What does detoxing feel like

No specific reactions noted

Further testing

Calcium, PTH and Vitamin D if barium is found elevated in a hair analyses.

Bismuth (Bi)

Nature of bismuth

There is no real personality to bismuth. Bismuth is a chemical element that is relatively non-toxic to humans when used in approved forms and at appropriate doses. Bismuth compounds, such as bismuth subsalicylate, are commonly used for their medicinal properties.

Role in the body

There is no significant physiological role in the body

Sources of bismuth

Bismuth compounds, in when combined with antibiotics, are used in the treatment of peptic ulcers associated with Helicobacter pylori infection. Bismuth helps to suppress the growth of H. pylori bacteria and promotes ulcer healing.

How to assess body burden

Urine is the best way to assess bismuth burden. It's important to note that bismuth compounds should be used as directed by healthcare professionals or according to the instructions on over-the-counter products. Bismuth should not be taken in excessive amounts or for prolonged periods without medical supervision.

If you have hold specific concerns about regarding bismuth or its effects potential impact on your health, it is recommended advisable to consult with a healthcare professional. They can provide accurate precise information and guidance based tailored on to your particular circumstances.

How bismuth affects health

Gastrointestinal Effects: Bismuth compounds, like bismuth subsalicylate, have protective and soothing properties on the gastrointestinal tract. They are often used to relieve symptoms of gastrointestinal conditions, such as diarrhoea, indigestion, and heartburn. Bismuth compounds can help reduce inflammation and provide a mild antimicrobial effect in the digestive system.

Stool Discolouration: When bismuth compounds are ingested, they can cause a temporary discolouration of the stool, turning it a dark or black colour. This effect is harmless and typically resolves after discontinuation of bismuth use.

Rare Allergic Reactions: Although rare, some individuals may experience allergic reactions to bismuth compounds. Allergic symptoms may include rash, itching, hives, swelling, and difficulty breathing. If any allergic reactions occur, medical attention should be sought immediately.

Neurological Effects: In very rare cases, excessive or prolonged exposure to high levels of bismuth (such as in certain occupational settings) can lead to neurotoxic effects. This can include symptoms such as headache, confusion, muscle weakness, tremors, and encephalopathy. However, such cases are extremely highly uncommon and typically associated with industrial exposure rather than normal use.

Toxicity symptoms

These are rare and would be associated with the affects mentioned above.

Protective measures

Avoid exposure where possible and support phase 2 detoxification when exposed.

Specific binders

No specific binders.

What does detoxing feel like

No specific reactions noted.

Further testing

No further testing unless the case requires it.

Boron (B)

The Nature of Boron

Boron has no specific personality, however; due to its impact on the sex hormones, often presents like menopause when needed.

Dosage considerations

12-20mg/day

Clinical indications

Steroid hormone modulation, bone health (osteoporosis), prostate cancer.

Role in the body:

Boron helps your body metabolise key vitamins and minerals.

It increases the production of oestrogen and testosterone.

Helps prevent osteoporosis and post-menopausal symptoms. Boron is best known for its role in bone health because of the effects on steroid hormones. Boron also markedly reduces urinary calcium and magnesium loss, as well as increases calcium absorption.

Modest boron supplementation has been shown to stimulate mitogen-activated protein kinases (MAPK), inducing cell proliferation and growth, however; aggressive boron supplementation has a paradoxical inhibitory effect on MAPK.

Boron supplementation increases half-life of available vitamin D, thereby minimising the onset of vitamin D deficiency symptoms.

Sources of boron

- Apples
- Coffee
- Grapes
- Leafy vegetables
- Legumes
- Nuts

How to assess boron need

Blood and urine boron measurements are used to establish supplementation efficacy, rates of excretion and dietary intake.

Hair can be used to screen for boron deficiency.

Symptoms associated with deficiency

Symptoms of boron deficiency are not fully known. Among the possible problems boron deficiency can cause include hyperthyroidism, imbalance of sex hormones, osteoporosis, arthritis and abnormalities in the function of the nervous system. Taking boron supplements by the mouth can help prevent deficiency.

Most associated symptom are those felt during menopause and include, hot flashes, and vaginal dryness and a higher risk of osteoporosis in post-menopausal women.

Symptoms associated with potential excess

Boron is not considered toxic. In animals, excessive intake affects calcium metabolism and may cause osteoporosis and increased urinary excretion of riboflavin.

Boron toxicity resulted in testicular atrophy, decreased seminal volume, decreased sexual activity and stunted growth.

Further testing

It may be useful to assess selenium, The selenium deficiency disease known as Kashin-Bek is associated with severe lack of boron (and other elements such as molybdenum and germanium). Boron is suspected as an aetiologic factor because Kashin-Bek disease produces a type of degenerative arthritis.

Assessing calcium and vitamin D along with a dual-energy X-ray absorptiometry (DXA) scan would be useful when assessing bone health.

You can also ask your healthcare provider if they have access to labs that assess bone resorption markers.

Cadmium (Cd)

The nature of cadmium

Cadmium's nature is that it creates bone pain that feels a lot like the pain of influenza. Cadmium also has a strong tendency very easily displaces zinc, so it can contribute to reduced immunity but also, lower testosterone or cause prostate issues in men. The principal organs most vulnerable to cadmium toxicity are the kidneys and lungs.

Role in the body

Cadmium is not regarded as essential to human life and is a toxic element.

Cadmium has an affinity to bind to the periosteum (the lining of the bones); this causes the bones to ache, which feels a lot like flu. Only a small amount of cadmium remains in the body after eating food contaminated with cadmium, but if consumed over a long period of time, cadmium can lead to kidney disease and cause bones to become weaker. Cadmium poisoning has been reported in many parts of the world. It is one of the global health problems that affect many organs. Long-term exposure to cadmium through air, water, soil, and food leads to cancer and organ system toxicity such as skeletal, urinary, reproductive, cardiovascular, central and peripheral nervous, and respiratory systems.

Cadmium and lead absorption is increased in iron-deficiency states, which may contribute to the associated neurotoxicity of both elements.

Sources of cadmium

Smoking cigarettes is the primary source. Ingestion of cadmium in food is the major principal source of cadmium for non-smokers. This metal is mostly mainly used in industries to produce paints, pigment alloys, coatings, batteries as well as plastics. Majority of cadmium, about three-fourths is used as an electrode component in producing alkaline batteries. Cadmium is emitted through industrial processes and from cadmium smelters into sewage sludge, fertilisers, and groundwater, which can remain in soils and sediments for several decades and be taken up by plants.

Therefore, significant human exposure to cadmium can be by the ingestion of contaminated foodstuffs, especially cereals, grains, fruits, and leafy vegetables as well as contaminated beverages. Also, people may get exposed to cadmium can by occur through inhalation through during the incineration of municipal waste.

Food grown on cadmium-contaminated soil - sewage sludge, fertilisers, and irrigation water can contaminate the soil, and have a knock-on effect on the following:

- Large ocean fish - tuna, cod, haddock
- Refined and processed foods
- Processed meats, cola drinks, and instant coffee
- Artists paints
- Air pollution - incineration of rubber tires, plastic, and paints
- Cigarette smoke
- Contaminated drinking water
- Occupational exposure - battery manufacture, semiconductors, dental materials
- Motor oil and exhaust fumes from cars
- Children today are commonly born with cadmium toxicity passed from mother to child via the placenta.

How to assess body burden

Cadmium levels can be measured in the blood, urine, and hair.

The best tests for assessing Cadmium are urine and hair. Although whole blood is useful for assessing acute or ongoing exposure, please note that blood levels drop very quickly after exposure.

How cadmium affects health

Blood - Iron deficiency anaemia has been reported in chronic cadmium toxicity.

Energy – cadmium causes potent inhibition of essential enzymes in the Krebs energy cycle.

Nervous System - cadmium inhibits the release of acetylcholine and activates cholinesterase. This results in a tendency for hyperactivity of the nervous system. Cadmium also directly damages nerve cells. induced metabolic and neurotransmitter alterations are also associated with GABA and serotonin. Even though the molecular basis of Cd neurotoxicity still needs to be fully unravelled, Cd intoxication could be relevant to AD, Parkinson's disease (PD), and Huntington's disease (HD).

Bones and Joints - cadmium alters calcium and phosphorus metabolism, thus contributing to arthritis, osteoporosis, and neuromuscular diseases.

Cardiovascular System - cadmium replaces zinc in the arteries, contributing to brittle, inflexible arteries. Cadmium chloride at 5 µM significantly inhibits angiogenesis, cellular migration, tube formation, and nitric oxide production, indicating that cadmium might impair endothelial functions by inhibiting endothelial nitric oxide synthase.

Digestive System - Cadmium is a toxic metal that can accumulate in a variety of crops, including spinach, potatoes, and many grains. While its toxicity extends beyond just the gastrointestinal tract, cadmium does exert a profound effect in that region. Cadmium can increase inflammatory gene expression in the epithelial cells lining the gut, which can subsequently lead to a disruption of the tight junctions that link these cells together. Predictably, with this disruption in gut integrity comes increases in permeability, allowing inflammatory molecules found in the gastrointestinal tract (such as LPS) to transgress the epithelial barrier and enter the bloodstream, increasing systemic inflammation. The good gut bacteria play a profound role in reducing cadmium toxicity, primarily via cadmium sequestration and subsequent elimination in faeces. Cadmium also interferes with the production of digestive enzymes that require zinc.

Male Reproductive System - prostate problems and impotence can result from cadmium-induced zinc deficiency.

Female Reproductive System (pregnancy) - Maternal exposure to Cd during pregnancy can result in a variety of adverse reproductive outcomes, such as maternal toxicity, placental damage/haemorrhage, impaired implantation, increased resorptions, reduced litter size, foetal growth retardation, congenital malformation in the foetus and embryonic/foetal death. Exposure to Cd during mid- to late gestation can result in both placental toxicity (reduced blood flow and necrosis) and diminished nutrient transport across the placenta. Exposure during the late gestation can also result in foetal death, despite low levels of Cd entering the foetus.

Endocrine System - zinc is required for growth and insulin release. Cadmium can contribute to failure to thrive, delayed growth development, and diabetes.

Excretory System -cadmium accumulates in the kidneys, resulting in high blood pressure and kidney disease.

Dental - alterations in calcium and vitamin D activity, caused by cadmium toxicity, can result in cavities and tooth deformities.

Psychological - cadmium toxicity is associated with learning disorders and hyperactivity. This may be due to zinc deficiency, or to inhibition of acetylcholine release in the brain.

Toxicity symptoms

The main symptoms include Femoral pain, lumbago, osteopenia, renal dysfunction, hypertension, vascular disease but can include anything from the lost below:

Alopecia (hair loss)	Failure to thrive syndrome
Anaemia	Fertility, decreased
Atherosclerosis	Hyperactivity in children
Arthritis (both osteo and rheumatoid)	Hypertension
Bone repair, inhibited	Hypoglycaemia
Cancer	Inflammation
Cerebral haemorrhage	Lung disease
Cholesterol, elevated	Migraine headaches
Cirrhosis of the liver	Osteoporosis
Diabetes	Renal (kidney) disease
Emphysema	Schizophrenia
Enlarged heart	Strokes
	Vascular disease

Protective measures

Avoid smoking as that is the main source. Reduce exposure to car exhaust fumes.

Support phase 2 detoxification.

Take the following nutrients:

- Zinc
- Iron

- Manganese
- Calcium
- Glutathione
- Alpha-lipoic acid
- Milk Thistle
- Garlic

Specific binders

EDTA, DMSA and NAC

Sacchyromyces boulardi

Chlorella

What does detoxing feel like

Due to the periosteum (lining of the bones) affinity, detoxing can feel like the bone pain you get from Flu. Other flu-like symptoms can occur as well.

Further testing

Iron and zinc stays should always be reassessed in relation to cadmium.

Calcium (Ca)

The nature of calcium

The nature of calcium as an element is hard and heavy – consider the oyster shell. It is not very active; it is hard and heavy. When there is too much calcium in our soft tissue, due to incorrect supplementation or, a lack of co-factors, or a hormonal imbalance, then the body starts to feel hard and heavy. Another way to describe a hard and heavy body is for that would be tired or fatigued.

Dosage considerations

Optimal forms of calcium include gluconate and citrate salts.

500 mg/d results in a significant rise in mean serum calcium and fall in serum alkaline phosphatase.

Clinical indications

Osteoporosis, hypertension

Role in the body

Calcium is essential for healthy bones and teeth, heart, nerves, muscles and blood clotting.

Calcium is extremely important to the human body. Not only is it vital for strong bones and teeth as well as muscle contractions, it but it also assists in muscle movement by carrying messages from the brain to all our body parts. Cells in all living things must communicate with, or "signal," one another. Calcium ions act as vital messengers between these cells and are necessary in all multicellular life forms. They also assist in the release of hormones and enzymes.

Calcium is nature's most renowned structural material. Indeed, calcium is a necessary component of all living things and is also abundant in many non-living things, particularly those that help support life, such as soil and water. Teeth, seashells (like the oyster shell), bones, and cave stalactites are all products of calcium. It is, however, also the most abundant metallic element in the human body, total-body calcium is about 980 grams, which is greater than any other element. The vast majority of calcium resides in bone.

The absorption of calcium relies on vitamin D, and the deposition of calcium, whether it goes into soft or hard tissue, relies on vitamin K. Magnesium is also necessary for proper assimilation and use of calcium in the body. In fact, if we take too much calcium and not enough magnesium, it can cause problems in the body. The metabolism of calcium is controlled by the thyroid and parathyroid glands. Calcium metabolism involves other nutrients, including protein and phosphorus.

A calcium imbalance can often look like an under-active thyroid and, in many cases, presents with the exact same symptoms! The reason for this is multi factorial but includes the role of calcium in cell membrane permeability. An excess of calcium in soft tissue interferes with cell membrane permeability, making it more difficult for hormones, such as thyroxine, to enter the cell. Thus, causing a functional hormone hormone-resistant state.

Blood levels are kept in a very strict range through various homeostatic mechanisms.

Although about 99% of our calcium is found in bone structures, calcium is essential for four other critical roles:

Cell Membrane Regulation - affecting cell permeability, T; the results of research suggest that the permeability of human cell membranes to sodium and potassium is regulated by internal calcium, which in turn is controlled by a calcium pump that utilises ATP (energy).

Body Fluid Regulation - Body Fluid Regulation – affecting Calcium affects blood clotting as well as, acidity, and alkalinity.

Regulation of cell division - Regulation of cell division. Calcium acts both to modulate intracellular signalling as a secondary messenger and to facilitate structural changes as cells progress through division.

Regulation of hormone secretion - Regulation of hormone secretion - insulin. Calcium ions stimulate insulin release into the blood. Thus, the higher the blood sugar concentration, the more insulin is released by beta-cells; an effect mediated by Calcium.

Functions Of Calcium

    Circulatory - excites the heart, constricts small blood vessels

    Excretory - inhibits water loss

    Digestive - in excess, is constipating

    Nervous - slows nerve impulse transmission

    Reproductive - required for normal cell division

Hormones - inhibits the release of thyroid-releasing and other pituitary hormones. It also plays a role in sugar metabolism and, diabetes.

Blood - stimulates blood formation and is required for blood clotting.

Muscular - Calcium triggers contraction in striated muscle. (A) Actomyosin in striated muscle. Striated muscle in the relaxed state has tropomyosin covering myosin-binding sites on actin. Calcium binds to troponin C, which induces a conformational change in the troponin complex. In other words, Calcium plays a very important role in muscles contracting.

Skeletal - Calcium is the main component of bone

Metabolic - required for phosphorus metabolism and energy production in the Krebs cycle

Detoxification - inhibits the uptake of lead and also, antagonises cadmium.

Cellular - decreases the permeability of cells to sodium and potassium ions

Sources of calcium

- Seafood - sardines, caviar, smelt and other small bony fish.
- Animal products - egg yolks and bone broth.
- Nuts/seeds - almonds, sesame seeds, hazelnuts.
- Vegetables - kale, collards, mustard greens, turnip greens
- Dairy - cheeses, milk
- Miscellaneous - molasses, kelp, brewer's yeast, torula yeast

How to assess need

Blood, hair or urine calcium, bone resorption markers, serum 25-hydroxyvitamin D, PTH and alkaline phosphatase.

Hair is an excellent way to assess overall calcium balance in relation to the other minerals. It is also a good indicator of hidden copper toxicity. There is a close relationship between high hair calcium and elevated tissue copper. This may be revealed on in the mineral analysis. Copper may be normal or even low in the hair because copper may accumulate in the liver or brain, but not in the hair. Some symptoms of a high calcium are due to copper imbalance.

These may include fatigue, depression, enhanced emotions, skin problems, spaciness, insomnia, or mind racing - and occasionally hyperthyroid symptoms.

In the latter, serum thyroxine levels may be elevated. Usually, the patient demonstrates only some of the symptoms of hyperthyroidism. This is because the excessive thyroid activity is secondary, due to a copper imbalance or to other factors. In addition to copper imbalance, low cell permeability may inhibit thyroid hormone from passing into the cells, and a low potassium level may diminish the sensitivity of the cells to thyroid hormone. These situations may cause the body to compensate by producing more thyroid hormone. Partial thyroidectomy or radioactive iodine therapy is usually not necessary if the biochemical imbalances are addressed. In these unusual cases, copper supplementation is often helpful. If you suspect copper to be imbalanced, please read that reference section next.

High calcium on a hair retest often means the body is eliminating excess calcium

A calcium urine test measures the amount of calcium in your urine. If your urine calcium levels are too high or too low, it may be a sign of kidney disease, kidney stones, bone disease, a parathyroid gland disorder, or other conditions.

Blood is unreliable unless the imbalance is seriously pathological. If you are using blood to monitor calcium, please also assess vitamin D, parathyroid and thyroid levels.

Symptoms associated with a calcium deficiency

- Alarm or fight-flight reaction
- Anxiety Irritability
- Bruising
- High blood pressure
- Insomnia
- Muscle cramps and spasms
- Nervousness
- Osteoporosis
- Tooth decay

Symptoms associated with a calcium excess

The main symptoms described with high calcium are weakness, lack of energy, poor appetite, nausea and vomiting, constipation, frequent urination, or abdominal or bone pain but can include any of the symptoms listed below:

- Apathy
- Arthritis
- Constipation
- Depression, mental
- Fatigue
- Gall stones
- Hardening of arteries
- Kidney stones
- Withdrawal, social

Nutrient relationships

Assist with absorption - vitamin A, and D, and protein. stomach acidity, protein in diet

Assist with utilisation - magnesium, copper, vitamin C, Vitamin K

Reduce absorption - fluoride, low stomach acidity, low protein in diet, phosphorus in excess

Reduce utilisation - lead, cadmium, sodium, potassium

Further testing

Since low albumin levels frequently, but not always, correspond to low calcium levels, albumin testing should always be included with serum calcium measurements.

Phosphate, creatinine, liver function tests, complete blood count, oestrogen, testosterone (in men), and thyroid-stimulating hormone can all be useful when assessing calcium.

When blood calcium drops, parathyroid hormone (PTH) is secreted to initiate osteoclastic activity. PTH also stimulates activation of vitamin D to calcitriol, increasing intestinal calcium absorption to assist PTH, so both PTH and vitamin D should be assessed.

Correcting a calcium imbalance also can involve support of adrenal and thyroid glandular activity, correction of copper imbalance, and correction of any other contributing causes.

Cesium (Cs)

Nature of Cesium:

Cesium is radioactive, its nature is to produce heat.

Role in the body

Cesium has no known beneficial role in the body.

Sources of cesium

You can be exposed to stable or radioactive cesium by breathing air, drinking water, or eating food containing cesium. The level of cesium in air and water is generally very low.

How to assess body burden

Laboratories use special techniques to measure the amount of cesium in body fluids such as blood and urine, as well as in faeces or other human samples. This can give an indication of whether a person has been exposed to levels of cesium that are higher than those normally found in food, water, or air.

Other radioactive metals that fall into this category and can be picked up in urine are Thallium, Thorium, and Uranium.

How cesium affects health

Cesium can have various effects on the body depending on the form and level of exposure. Here's an overview of how cesium can affect the body:

Radioactive Cesium-137: The radioactive isotope cesium-137 is a byproduct of nuclear fission, commonly found in nuclear power plants and nuclear fallout. If ingested or inhaled in significant amounts, cesium-137 can emit ionising radiation, which poses a significant health risk. Ionising radiation can damage cells and DNA, leading to an increased risk of cancer and other radiation-related illnesses. Exposure is very rare.

Non-Radioactive Cesium: Non-radioactive cesium, such as naturally occurring cesium-133, is generally considered to have low toxicity. The body can naturally eliminate non-radioactive cesium through urine. However, ingestion of large amounts of non-radioactive cesium can still cause adverse effects.

Gastrointestinal Effects: Ingestion of large amounts of cesium can irritate the gastrointestinal tract, leading to symptoms such as nausea, vomiting, diarrhoea, and abdominal pain. These effects are primarily associated with high doses or excessive consumption.

Cardiovascular Effects: Cesium can interfere with the electrical signalling of the heart and affect heart rhythm. Ingestion or exposure to high levels of cesium can lead to cardiac arrhythmias, which can potentially be life-threatening. However, significant cardiovascular effects are typically associated with exposure to high concentrations or radioactive forms of cesium.

It's important to note that cesium is not commonly encountered in everyday environments or in at levels that would pose significant health risks. Exposure to significant amounts of cesium-137 is primarily a concern in situations involving nuclear accidents, nuclear waste mishandling, or occupational settings involving radioactive materials.

If you have concerns about exposure or suspect exposure to any radioactive element, it is crucial to seek immediate medical attention and follow the guidance of healthcare professionals and relevant authorities. They can provide appropriate assessment, monitoring, and treatment specific to your situation.

Toxicity symptoms

High levels of radioactive cesium in or near your body can cause nausea, vomiting, diarrhoea, bleeding, coma, and even death.

Protective measures

In a radiation emergency, some people may be told to take potassium iodide (KI) to protect their thyroid. Do not take KI unless instructed by public health or emergency response officials or a healthcare provider. There are limits to who should use KI and how much it can help.

People over age 40 have a low risk of developing radiation-induced thyroid cancer, so they may need a smaller dose than younger people or may not need to take potassium iodide at all.

The risk is higher in children and infants. As a result, children and infants will likely need to take potassium iodide. It's safe for these age groups when taken at the proper dose.

In an emergency, public health officials will determine which age groups should take the medication.

Specific binders

No specific binders.

What does detoxing feel like

No specific reactions noted.

Further testing

No further testing unless the case requires it.

Chromium (Cr)

The nature of chromium

Chromium slaps your hand when you reach for that extra piece of cake. It is involved in regulating blood sugar and cravings and plays a vital role in regulating insulin.

Dosage considerations

Optimal forms include nicotinate, chloride, histidine or picolinate salts.

Chromium picolinate (200–100 µg) is an effective supplementation for treating diabetes and weight gain from insulin insensitivity.

Clinical indications

Blood sugar dys-regulatory conditions

Role in the body

Chromium is important in the breakdown of fats and carbohydrates. It stimulates fatty acid and cholesterol synthesis. They are important for brain function and other body processes. Chromium also aids in insulin action and glucose breakdown.

Unlike most essential elements that have multiple metabolic functions, the only known role for chromium (Cr) is in potentiating insulin receptor tyrosine kinase. It is the main ingredient of Glucose tolerance factor.

Other possible roles involved in the synthesis of DNA as well as the functions listed below.

Circulatory - serum cholesterol regulation

Digestive - sugar and carbohydrate utilisation (via insulin)

Nervous - maintenance of nervous system by regulation of blood sugar

Eyes - corneal clarity

Muscular - supplies energy for muscular contraction

Skeletal - essential component of bones and hair

Protective - immune system (via insulin)

Metabolic - fat, protein, and carbohydrate metabolism regulation

Sources of chromium

- Seafood - oysters
- Meats - calves' liver, egg yolk
- Nuts/seeds - peanuts
- Fruit - grape juice
- Dairy - American cheese
- Grains - wheat and wheat germ
- Miscellaneous - brewer's yeast, black pepper, molasses

How to assess need

Inductively coupled plasma mass spectrographic (ICP-MS) methods allow accurate detection of chromium in urine, serum and whole blood. Insulin and blood glucose can also be used to assess chromium need. Given the difficulties with interpretation of direct chromium concentration measurements, functional evidence for dysglycaemia, such as elevated blood glucose and insulin levels, or an abnormal glucose-insulin tolerance test can provide a functional assessment of chromium insufficiency.

Urine excretion may reflect recent intake, while circulating serum chromium may not be in equilibrium with biologically active stores. Hair levels are thought to suggest past fluctuations in chromium intake.

A high chromium level in a hair analysis is often indicative of a loss of chromium through the hair and is frequently caused by an iron toxicity or another mineral imbalance problem. Assess Iron in blood

High blood and urine chromium can be from supplementation

Hair results correlate to a functional need, supplementing with chromium when the chromium reading is low, is frequently helpful in correcting symptoms of fatigue, or sugar and carbohydrate intolerance.

Excessive iron intake is a frequent cause of both high and low chromium levels. Assess accordingly.

Symptoms associated with deficiency

- Atherosclerosis
- Blood sugar conditions (diabetes and hypoglycaemia)
- Depressed growth
- Elevated serum cholesterol levels
- Fatigue
- Neurodegenerative or memory disorders

Symptoms associated with potential excess

- Asthma
- Allergies
- Calcium deficiency
- Diarrhoea
- Iron deficiency
- Kidney damage
- Sinusitis
- Ulcers
- Vomiting

Nutrient relationships

Synergistic Nutrients - magnesium, vitamin B6, zinc, manganese

Reduces absorption - iron, manganese, zinc, vanadium, phytates

Further testing

Insulin, glucose, HbA1C to rule out any effects on glucose metabolism.

Cobalt (Co)

The nature of cobalt

Cobalt, in the right quantities, soothes the nervous system and gives energy when needed. Cobalt is an essential component of vitamin B12, which is necessary for the proper function of cells and, the production of red blood cells, and maintaining the Myelin sheath that covers nerves.

Dosage considerations

Intake of 1.5 µg/d of vitamin B12 supplies about 0.06 µg cobalt.

Clinical indications

B12 deficiency or pernicious anaemia

Role in the body

Cobalt is only functional in the body as part of vitamin B-12. It's needed for making red blood cells (erythropoiesis), nerve maintenance as well as thyroid function. Cobalt has some of the same jobs as manganese and zinc. It can replace manganese in by activating several of the same enzymes that need manganese.

Needed for the formation of vitamin B12 - blood formation, nervous system protection.

Sources of cobalt

- Meats
- Liver
- Fish
- Nutritional yeast
- Nuts
- Green leafy vegetables Some cereals
- Vegetarians may have a deficiency of this mineral since fruits and vegetables contain no cobalt except for cabbage, legumes, spinach, lettuce, figs, and turnips.

How to assess need

Whole blood, urine and hair.

Symptoms associated with deficiency

- Pernicious anaemia (deficiency of vitamin B12).
- The common symptoms due to acute cobalt deficiency are tingling of hands or feet, paleness, weakness, fatigue, loss of appetite, weight loss, and subsequent poor growth, shortness of breath, dizziness, scaly ears, and watery discharge from the eyes.

Symptoms associated with potential excess

- Excess red blood cell formation
- Cardiomyopathy
- Dermatitis
- Goitre

Nutrient relationships

B12 and folate

Further testing

Assess B12 needs if cobalt is low

Copper (Cu)

The nature of copper

Copper is a blessing and a curse, depending on its balance.

Copper is the 'female' of the periodic table, zinc being the 'male'. Copper can be a bit of a bitch when she is out of balance in either direction... too much and she makes you cry for no reason, have uncontrolled thoughts and gives you sharp headaches. Too little, and you fall apart physically more than mentally! At her best, she is loving, kind, and nurturing, at her worst she is psychotic!

Dosage considerations

Aspartate or sulphate salts are the best forms.

Clinical indications

Refractory anaemia, depigmentation, impaired glucose tolerance, cardiac-related problems, elevated cholesterol.

Role in the body

There is a lot of focus on copper excess and very little on deficiency, but they are both relevant.

There is a strong correlation between copper and oestrogen. Copper toxicity and excess copper levels causes the body to hold onto oestrogen in the body and prevent its detoxification, and having excess oestrogen levels and poor oestrogen detoxification causes the body to hold onto copper. They tend to feed one another, creating a vicious cycle. Copper stimulates oestrogen production, and oestrogen can increase copper in the body; they, too, are very connected. When one goes up, the other can follow. This effect can be seen in both genders.

We can become copper-toxic in a variety of ways. Hormonal birth control (pill, patch, ring), copper pipes, copper IUDs, and hormone replacement therapy. It can even be something that was passed to you in-utero from your mother. The symptoms of excess copper are very similar to oestrogen dominance. Copper is predominantly deposited in the brain and liver. In our homes, copper conducts electricity. It does something similar in the brain. One of the main features of excess copper in the brain is the occurrence of abhorrent thoughts

(thoughts not normal to the personality), moodiness, and, very commonly, weepiness over the smallest triggers. A It's a lot like the symptoms experienced by a women woman experiencing PMS!

Many of the most prevalent metabolic dysfunctions of our time are related in some way to a copper imbalance. Copper toxicity is a much much-overlooked contributor to many health problems; including severe mental health disorders, anorexia, fatigue, premenstrual syndrome, depression, anxiety, migraine headaches, allergies, childhood hyperactivity, and learning disorders. Copper plays a role in all the elements listed below:

- Energy production
- Female reproductive system
- Blood formation
- Formation of melanin and keratin.
- Synthesis of connective tissue and myoglobin.
- Haemoglobin synthesis (incorporation of iron into haemoglobin).
- Energy production (the electron transport system).
- Synthesis of neurotransmitters (the catecholamines).
- Free radical scavenging (superoxide dismutase).
- Retention of calcium in the bone matrix.
- Immune system (control of anaerobic organisms) and formation of reticuloendothelial cells.
- Formation of the myelin sheath of nerves.
- Fertility and maintenance of pregnancy.

Functions Of Copper

Circulatory - structure of blood vessels, aorta, and heart muscle

Blood - formation of haemoglobin

Nervous - maintenance of the myelin sheath on nerves

Reproductive - essential for fertility, menstrual cycle

Endocrine - synthesis of stimulatory neurotransmitters

Muscular/skeletal - bone and connective tissue structure

Immune system - necessary for the immune system

Integumentary - needed for skin, hair, nails and pigments

Energy - energy production (the electron transport system)

Sources Of Copper

This is a heavy metal which that is used in industries to produce copper pipes, cables, wires, copper cookware, etc. It is also used to make copper intrauterine devices and birth control pills. Copper in the form of copper sulphate is added to drinking water and swimming pools. Due to our history of industrial activities, it can accumulate in the soil and up be taken by plants. As such, copper is present in some nuts, avocados, wheat germ and bran, and other foods.

Main sources include:

- **Seafood** - oysters, crabs, bluefish, perch, lobster
- **Meats** - veal, duck, lamb, pork, beef liver and kidneys
- **Nuts/seeds** - cashews, almonds, pecans, walnuts, brazil nuts, sesame seeds, sunflower seeds, pistachios
- **Vegetables** - soybeans
- **Grains** - wheat germ and bran
- **Miscellaneous** - yeast, gelatine, bone meal, corn oil, margarine, mushrooms, chocolate
- **Other sources** -Copper plumbing was hailed as a great advance in the 1940's and today, many homes still have copper plumbing. Copper can be leached from pipes, especially in areas with acidic water, leaving, in severe cases, a greenish ring on bathroom fixtures. Water coolers and icemakers in refrigerators also use copper tubing. Water that sits in these units can contain dangerously high levels of copper.

Copper Cookware. Copper tea kettles and other copper cookware can be a source of copper toxicity if used frequently over a period, especially when cooking acidic foods like tomatoes.

Drinking Water Contaminated with Copper. High amounts of naturally occurring copper can occur in water supplies. Also, copper sulphate is added to some municipal drinking water supplies to kill yeast and fungi.

Birth Control Pills and Copper Intrauterine Devices. One of the side effects of the birth control pill is that it tends to raise copper levels in the body. This is due to the close association between the hormone oestrogen and copper levels. Several hundred milligrams of copper a year can easily be absorbed from a copper IUD. These devices can be very harmful for women prone to high copper levels, especially if they are deficient in zinc and/or iron.

Vitamin and Mineral Supplements. Copper is frequently added to vitamin supplements, particularly prenatal vitamins. Although this is a benefit for some people, it can be harmful for many other women. I would advise assessing copper before supplementing it.

Fungicides for Swimming Pools and Foods. Copper sulphate is added to swimming pools and may be sprayed on fruits and vegetables to retard the growth of algae and fungus.

Vegetarianism and Other High-Copper Diets. Many diets today are high in copper. In particular, vegetarian proteins such as soybeans, nuts, seeds, tofu, avocados, and grains are high in copper content. The high fibre in vegetables can also decrease the absorption of zinc, which is needed to balance copper.

Other high-copper foods are organ meats, shellfish, wheat germ and bran, yeast, corn oil, margarine, and mushrooms.

Occupational Exposure. Plumbers, welders, machinists, and others who work with copper are at risk for copper toxicity.

Dental Appliances. Copper is used in dental alloys in fillings, crowns, and other appliances.

Adrenal Gland Exhaustion and Copper Toxicity. Other than hormone replacement therapies involving oestrogen, diminished adrenal activity is perhaps the single most important physiological reason for copper problems today. The reason is that adrenal activity is required to stimulate the production of ceruloplasmin, the primary copper-binding protein. When adrenal activity is insufficient, ceruloplasmin synthesis in the liver declines.

Copper that is not bound cannot be used, and unbound copper begins to accumulate in various tissues and organs.

Zinc Deficiency and Copper Toxicity. A widespread zinc deficiency in our population is another critical cause of a copper imbalance. Zinc and copper normally exist in a delicate balance. Zinc is a primary copper antagonist. When zinc is deficient, copper tends to accumulate in various storage organs.

Congenital Copper Imbalance. Mothers deficient in zinc, or high in copper, transmit these imbalances to their children through the placenta. Mothers also pass on to their children other nutrient deficiencies and toxic metals, which impair the child's adrenal glands. Weak adrenal glands, in turn, results in a worsening of the copper imbalance in the child by the mechanism explained above. Many children are born these days with excessive copper levels passed to them from their mothers in utero.

Mould exposure. Moulds and mycotoxin exposure, especially to the Fusarium mould species and a mycotoxin called Zearanolone, can also cause copper to be retained by the body.

How to assess need:

Copper deficiency: RBC Cu, Serum ceruloplasmin, elevated urinary HVA:VMA ratio, bone resorption markers

Copper excess: urine and hair

Blood Tests - Copper and ceruloplasmin levels can be measured in serum to detect copper poisoning. There will be some daily fluctuations, as with all blood tests, but this is a useful measure. Unfortunately, few physicians run these tests routinely.

Increased blood and normal or increased ceruloplasmin concentration may indicate exposure to excess copper or may be associated with conditions that decrease copper excretion – such as liver disease.

Hair Analysis - Hair analysis is a rapid, simple screening test that can reveal both direct and hidden copper imbalance. A copper level exceeding 2.50 mg% is considered elevated. However, there are several readings that indicate hidden copper toxicity. In other words, copper may not show up high on the hair test but may be stored in various organs and will show up later as it is mobilised.

Hair Analysis - Often copper status can be tricky to assess. Copper may be present, but unavailable for use in the body. This occurs any time adrenal gland activity is low.

Hidden Copper Toxicity can exist. Copper is often normal on hair tests but may be locked in body tissues. Test indicators of a hidden copper imbalance are:

- Calcium level greater than 75 mg%
- Potassium level less than 3 mg%
- Sodium/potassium ratio less than 2.2:1
- Mercury toxicity often indicates a hidden copper toxicity
- Copper level less than 1.0 mg%
- Zinc/copper ratio less than 6:1

Urine testing: Increased blood and urine copper concentrations and normal or increased ceruloplasmin concentration may indicate exposure to excess copper or may be associated with conditions that decrease copper excretion – such as liver disease. Increased hepatic copper may be present with chronic conditions.

You can use the checklist on the next page to assess for hidden copper in a hair analysis and match the results with the symptoms.

Symptoms associated with potential excess:

Acne	Headaches, Migraines
Allergies	Hyperactivity
Alopecia	Hypertension
Anaemia	Hypoglycaemia
Anxiety	Hypothyroidism
Arthritis	Iron Storage Disease
Atherosclerosis	Liver Detoxification and Dysfunction
Autism	Oestrogen levels elevated
Candida Albicans (Yeast) Infections	Premenstrual Tension & PMDD
Cholesterol elevation	Psychosis
Depression	Schizophrenia
Diabetes	Tooth Decay
'Failure To Thrive' Syndrome	Urinary Tract Infection

On the next page is a useful tool when assessing copper through a hair analysis, you want as few Yes's as possible! Anything over 10 and you potentially have hidden copper toxicity.

Copper elevated or < 1	Yes / No
Calcium elevated	Yes / No
Magnesium elevated	Yes / No
Potassium < 4	Yes / No
Zinc very low or very high	Yes / No
Mercury elevated	Yes / No
Ca:P > 10:1	Yes / No
Phosphorus < 12	Yes / No
Molybdenum low	Yes / No
Na:K , 2.2:1 or elevated	Yes / No
Cry often or for no reason	Yes / No
Premenstrual syndrome in women	Yes / No
Acne around jaw line	Yes / No
Hair loss	Yes / No
Easy bruising	Yes / No
White spots on nails	Yes / No

But copper is not all bad all the time... in fact in the right balance, copper is an essential nutrient!

Symptoms associated with deficiency:

Anaemia	Hair loss
Atherosclerosis	Impaired collagen formation
Demyelination of nerves	Loss of hair colour
Fatigue	Low hormone production
Oedema	Osteoporosis
Diarrhoea	Hot flushes

Nutrient relationships

Always consider N-Acetyl cysteine and other antioxidants when working with excess copper.

Calcium and copper have an affinity to each other in that they tend to both be low or high together, assess accordingly.

Zinc, manganese, iron, calcium, molybdenum, sulphur, Vitamin B6, vitamin C all lower the levels of copper.

Mercury and Cadmium can also lower copper and should be assessed if the levels are low.

High levels of vitamin C inhibits the absorption of copper, possibly through increasing iron absorption, which is a copper antagonist.

Copper, in excess, tends to lower manganese, zinc, and potassium levels. Copper toxicity can also result in a deficiency of vitamin C and B6, inositol, folic acid, and rutin.

Copper tends to increase tissue levels of calcium and sodium.

Copper can displace iron from the liver.

Mercury, cadmium, and zinc – compete for absorption.

Molybdenum and sulphur – bind copper in the intestine.

Iron and manganese – remove copper from the liver.

Zinc – lowers copper levels in the blood.

Vitamin C – chelates copper in the blood.

Vitamin B6, folic acid and niacin are also copper antagonists.

Cobalt is synergistic with copper.

Further testing

Oestrogen and adrenal status

Additional information considering copper can be both nutritionally beneficial OR toxic:

Restore Adrenal Activity

Restore normal adrenal gland activity through nutrition, adaptogenic herbs, and positive lifestyle changes. A reduction in stressful activity is advisable. Adequate rest, sleep, and avoiding excessive exercise is beneficial. Nutritional supplement programs to enhance adrenal activity should include vitamins C and E, manganese, pantothenic acid, and, in some cases, adrenal glandular substances. Specific dosages depend on individual cases.

What it feels like to detox

During the correction of a copper imbalance, copper elimination frequently causes transient symptoms, including weepiness (for no reason), headaches, skin rash, free-floating anxiety, insomnia, fatigue, and a flare-up of chronic conditions related to a copper imbalance. These reactions generally last a day or two but can last 4 four days and then subside. The supplement program may be temporarily reduced if a symptom becomes particularly annoying. These symptoms are indications of a healing process and should be welcomed!

Dietary Considerations

Copper-toxic individuals have a great need to increase their protein intake, but usually will not partake of an increased meat protein intake until their adrenal insufficiency problem is improved or corrected. Until such time, the copper-toxic individual must avail him or herself of digestive aids, including hydrochloric acid and pancreatic enzymes.

One of the major problems associated with a copper toxicity problem is a copper-induced protein deficiency. This no doubt occurs, in part, because an excess of tissue copper causes a zinc deficiency. Adding to the problem, individuals suffering from copper toxicity frequently develop a distaste for meat protein due to their reduced ability to digest and assimilate protein. Over time, a serious protein deficiency develops. As stated previously, one major reason why copper accumulates in the body is a deficiency of protein required to bind copper. Although sometimes difficult, copper-toxic individuals should attempt to increase their protein intake (eggs, fish, or chicken). Soy-protein products should be avoided, unless otherwise specified, if possible, as soy products contain relatively high amounts of copper.

An adequate level of zinc, so necessary to prevent an excessive copper buildup, depends largely on the eating of red meat protein. As stated previously, individuals suffering from copper toxicity develop a strong aversion to the eating of zinc-rich red meat protein, hence the tendency to the excessive accumulation of tissue copper.

Fluoride (Fl)

Nature of fluoride

Although fluoride can, in tiny doses, benefit your teeth, higher doses can negatively impact the brain as well as impede certain enzymes. As a molecule that resembles iodine, it can also affect thyroid hormones and has been implicated it neurological issues.

Role in the body

Dental Health: Fluoride is most recognised for its role in preventing and reversing dental caries (tooth decay) and building strong teeth and bones. It inhibits or reverses the initiation and progression of dental caries and stimulates new bone formation.

Bone Health: Fluoride in trace amounts is essential for normal bone growth. It stimulates bone-building cells called osteoblasts and hormones such as insulin-like growth factor. A chronic deficiency, especially in children, can lead to weak or brittle bones.

It's important to note that excessive fluoride intake can lead to negative effects, such as dental fluorosis, skeletal fluorosis, cognitive impairment, and enzyme and electrolyte derangement. However, these negative effects are typically associated with excessive intake or prolonged high exposure. It's recommended to consult with dental and healthcare professionals for personalised advice on fluoride use and to ensure that fluoride intake is appropriate for your specific needs and circumstances. There is a recipe for non-fluoridated, homemade toothpaste in the eBook. You can use this on alternative days to reduce your exposure to fluoride in toothpaste. Please ensure you always spit out and rinse off any excess toothpaste!

Sources of fluoride

- Toothpaste and mouth washes
- Fluoridated water is found in most community water systems.
- Some foods and beverages naturally contain fluoride, although in varying amounts. Examples include brewed black tea and coffee, as the plants absorb fluoride from the soil.
- Grapes and raisins are also natural sources of fluoride.

- Additionally, certain fruits and vegetables, such as apples, strawberries, bananas, peaches, spinach, and potatoes, may contain fluoride
- Seafood, such as shrimp and crab legs, can be a natural source of fluoride.
- Processed foods made with fluoridated water may also contribute to fluoride intake.
- Some medications can also contain fluoride.

How to assess body burden

Fluoride concentrations can be measured in plasma, saliva, and urine to assess total fluoride exposure. These measures can provide information on fluoride circulating in the body. It's important to note that criteria for adequate, high, or low levels of fluoride in the body have not been established. Additionally, fluoride levels can vary depending on factors such as water source, diet, and geographic location.

How fluoride affects health

Tooth discolouration, tooth decay, endemic skeletal fluorosis (join and bone weakness). Exposure to fluoride before birth could lead to poorer cognitive outcomes in the future. Higher levels of fluoride lead to low scores in IQ tests.

There is a significant correlation between high blood pressure and water with too much fluoride.

Regular intake of fluoride may lead fluoroderma which results in acne and painful sores.

There may also be an increased risk of seizures.

Toxicity symptoms

Acne

Tooth discolouration and decay

Seizures

Weak joints

Protective measures

To remove excess fluoride from the body, here are some strategies that can be considered:

Stop consuming fluoride: The first step is to reduce or eliminate the intake of fluoride from various sources, such as fluoridated toothpaste, mouthwash, and dental products. Switching to fluoride-free alternatives can help minimise further exposure.

Drink filtered water: Reverse osmosis water filtration systems can effectively remove fluoride from tap water. Using reverse osmosis water or water that has been filtered by any methods, for drinking and cooking can help reduce fluoride intake.

Increase iodine intake: Iodine has been suggested to assist in the detoxification of fluoride from the body. Foods rich in iodine, such as seaweed, vegetables, cabbage, chicken eggs, and potatoes, can be incorporated into the diet to support this process.

Support detoxification: Consuming a nutrient-rich diet that supports overall detoxification can be beneficial. This includes eating a variety of fruits, vegetables, and whole foods, as well as staying hydrated to support the body's natural detoxification processes.

It's important to note that the body can naturally eliminate fluoride over time. However, the specific duration may vary depending on individual factors such as overall health, exposure levels, and the presence of other minerals in the body.

If you have concerns about fluoride exposure or suspect excessive fluoride intake, it's recommended to consult with a healthcare professional for personalised advice and guidance.

Specific binders

No specific binders

What does detoxing feel like

No specific symptoms noted

Further testing

No further testing unless the case requires it, e.g.: Thyroid function.

Gadolinium (Gd)

The nature of gadolinium

There is no notable nature to gadolinium.

Role in the body

Has no know physiological benefit. There is no known role in the body other than as an MRI contrast material.

Sources of gadolinium

MRI contrast scans, either directly through having a scan or through water contamination. Gadolinium accumulation in aquatic environments is concerning. High levels of administered GBCAs are excreted in urine and flushed down the toilet, especially at hospitals. Gadolinium is only partially removed during water treatment, and there is concern that the treatment process may de-chelate gadolinium from its ligand.

How to assess body burden

Urine is the best method of assessing exposure.

Natural gadolinium exposure is very rare and most people that have never received a GBCA will only show trace levels in urine. Urine is the best marker for gadolinium as it is primarily excreted via the kidneys, and because it is rapidly cleared from blood circulation, so blood levels are not a good indicator of gadolinium retention in the body. Urine gadolinium levels are very high after GBCA administration, and gradually drop close to zero after many years. Gadolinium excretion is highly correlated with the time passed since the last GBCA administration, but some people excrete it faster or slower than others.

How gadolinium affects health

Free gadolinium (Gd^{3+}) is a very toxic heavy metal because its ionic radius is very similar to that of calcium. Free gadolinium can block calcium channels and inhibit nerve transmissions, muscle contraction, blood coagulation, and mitochondrial function. Gadolinium can also replace calcium in bone. In fact, the sample on the next page is taken from a case of chronic progressing osteoporosis.

Gadolinium is a rare-earth heavy metal that most humans should have very little exposure to. It has a very common medical use: gadolinium-based contrast agents (GBCAs). GBCAs were first approved in 1988 to help make diseased tissues look brighter or darker during Magnetic Resonance Imaging (MRI). In 2017, nearly 40% of MRIs used GBCAs, and it is estimated that over 450 million GBCAs have been administered worldwide since 1988. While most gadolinium is flushed from the body following an MRI exam, new research suggests extended retention in multiple organs, leading to potential health issues. It is now also suspected to have contaminated water in the areas it is used in as water filtration doesn't filter it well before returning it to our drinking water sources.

While gadolinium itself is considered relatively safe, there have been concerns about its long-term effects and the potential for a condition known as gadolinium deposition disease (GDD).

Gadolinium Deposition Disease (GDD): GDD is a condition characterised by the accumulation of gadolinium in body tissues, even after the administration of GBCAs. It primarily affects individuals with impaired kidney function, as the kidneys play a crucial role in filtering and excreting gadolinium from the body. Symptoms of GDD may include persistent pain in the bones, joints, or skin, cognitive difficulties, skin thickening or discolouration, and other systemic symptoms. However, it's important to note that GDD is considered rare, and the majority of patients who receive GBCAs do not develop this condition.

Nephrogenic Systemic Fibrosis (NSF): NSF is another rare but serious condition associated with gadolinium exposure. It occurs primarily in individuals with pre-existing kidney problems and is characterised by the development of excessive fibrous tissue in the skin, joints, and other organs. The use of certain types of GBCAs has been strongly linked to NSF, especially in patients with severe renal impairment.

Gadolinium Retention: Research has shown that even in individuals with normal kidney function, small amounts of gadolinium can be retained in the body following GBCA administration. The long-term effects of gadolinium retention are not yet fully understood, and ongoing studies are being conducted to determine its potential health implications. However, it's important to note that the clinical significance of this retention is still a subject of debate among medical experts.

To mitigate potential risks associated with gadolinium exposure, medical professionals follow guidelines for GBCA use, particularly in patients with impaired kidney function. They carefully consider the risk-benefit ratio and utilise the lowest necessary dose of gadolinium for each patient.

Toxicity symptoms

These are rare and are associated with the health impacts listed above. Acute Adverse Effects: When administered as a contrast agent, gadolinium can cause immediate, transient side effects in some individuals, including headache, nausea, dizziness, and a metallic taste in the mouth. However, these effects are generally mild and short-lived.

Protective measures

Filter your water

Specific binders

No specific binders are noted

What does detoxing feel like

No specific symptoms are noted

Further testing

None unless the case requires it

Iodine (I)

Nature of iodine

Iodine is protective and nourishing.

It helps by providing energy and supporting metabolism and neurological health as well as protecting against cancer and even radiation.

Iodine is an essential nutrient for thyroid hormones and energy but is best kept in balance!

Dosage considerations

Although up to 1,000 µg of iodine daily is considered safe, therapeutic doses of iodine are not agreed upon, making iodine testing very important when it comes to patient care. Iodine repletion doses range between 90 µg/d and 50mg depending on the case. Consider food options first.

If you are concerned about the safety of supplementing iodine you can soak your feet in a foot bath that has a cap full of provolone iodine and epsom salts. Your body will absorb what it needs and there is no risk of overdosing.

Clinical indications

Goitre, hypothyroidism, hyperthyroidism, fibrocystic breast disease

Role in the body

Here are some of the roles of iodine in the body:

Thyroid Hormone Production: Iodine is necessary to produce thyroid hormones, which regulate many important biochemical reactions in the body, including protein synthesis and enzymatic activity. Thyroid hormones are critical determinants of metabolic activity and play a role in growth and development.

Brain Development: Iodine is important for foetal and infant brain development. Adequate iodine intake during pregnancy and infancy is essential for proper brain development and can help prevent intellectual disability.

Bone Health: Iodine is important for bone health and development. It plays a role in the regulation of calcium and phosphorus metabolism, which are important for bone growth and maintenance.

Immune System Functioning: Iodine is important for immune system functioning. It helps support the body's natural defence mechanisms against infections and diseases. As a topical it is antiseptic and ant fungal.

Breast Health: Iodine is important for breast health and may help reduce the risk of breast cancer. It plays a role in the regulation of oestrogen metabolism and can help prevent fibrocystic breast disease.

It's important to note that iodine deficiency can lead to negative effects, such as stunted growth, intellectual disability, and an enlarged thyroid gland (goitre). However, excessive iodine intake can also be harmful and can cause thyroid gland inflammation and thyroid cancer. It's recommended to consult with healthcare professionals for personalised advice on iodine intake and to ensure that iodine intake is appropriate for your specific needs and circumstances.

Sources of iodine

- Seaweed: Seaweed is one of the best food sources of iodine. Different types of seaweed, such as kelp, nori, kombu, and wakame, contain varying amounts of iodine.
- Fish and Seafood: Fish and seafood are good sources of iodine. Cod, tuna, shrimp, oysters, and other shellfish are particularly good sources.
- Dairy Products: Dairy products, such as milk, cheese, and yogurt, contain iodine. In general, the iodine content of dairy products is influenced by the iodine content of the animal feed.
- Eggs: Eggs are a good source of iodine. One hard-boiled egg provides about 26 mcg of iodine.
- Enriched Bread: Some bread manufacturers add iodate dough conditioner to their bread to enrich the iodine content.
- Fruits and Vegetables: Most fruits and vegetables are poor sources of iodine, but some contain small amounts. The iodine content of fruits and vegetables is influenced by the iodine content of the soil where they are grown.

- It's important to note that the iodine content of foods can vary depending on factors such as soil composition and agricultural practices. Additionally, iodine levels can vary depending on the geographic location and dietary habits of the individual.

How to assess need

There are several methods to assess iodine levels in the body. Here are some of the most used methods:

Urinary Iodine Concentration (UIC): UIC is a reliable biomarker of recent iodine intake for the population. The kidneys excrete approximately 90% of ingested iodine, and UIC from spot samples can provide information on recent iodine intake. A median 24-hour iodine urine collection is the best diagnostic test to identify iodine deficiency in a population.

Thyroid Volume: Assessment of thyroid volume can be used to monitor iodine sufficiency in a population. Thyroid volume can be measured using ultrasound or other imaging techniques.

Thyroid function tests: Good tests include urinary iodine, TSH, TT4, TT3, FT4, FT3, RT3

Dried Whole-Blood Spot Thyroglobulin (Tg) Levels: Dried whole-blood spot thyroglobulin (Tg) levels can be used to assess iodine status in populations. Tg is a protein produced by the thyroid gland, and its levels can be used as an indicator of iodine status.

Serum Iodine Concentration: Blood serum iodine concentration can be used to assess iodine status in populations. It reflects recent iodine intake and can be used to monitor iodine sufficiency in populations.

Dietary Questionnaires: Dietary questionnaires can be used to estimate iodine intake in populations. However, this method is the least reliable and may not accurately reflect actual iodine intake.

Functional Iodine Tests: The iodine skin test is a traditional approximation method of checking iodine status by painting the skin with a solution of iodine

Iodine patch test: The iodine patch test is a test where doctors paint a patch of iodine on your skin and check how it looks 24 hours later. This test is inexpensive and relatively quick but may not be as accurate as others.

It's important to note that no test can reliably diagnose iodine deficiency in individual patients. Additionally, iodine levels can vary depending on factors such as water source, diet, and geographic location. It's recommended to consult with healthcare professionals for personalised advice on iodine intake and to ensure that iodine intake is appropriate for your specific needs and circumstances.

Symptoms associated with deficiency

- Constipation
- Depression
- Difficulty concentrating
- Dry skin
- Enlarged thyroid or goiter
- Feeling cold
- Hair loss
- Serve tiredness and muscle weakness
- Thick puffy skin or puffiness of the face
- Unexpected weight gain
- Weak, slow heartbeat

Symptoms associated with potential excess

Excessive intake of iodine reduces organic binding of iodine, resulting in hypothyroidism and goitre, thyroiditis, and autonomous thyroid nodules.

Excessive iodine intake can also stimulate autoimmune thyroiditis

Nutrient relationships

Biotin can affect thyroid test results, please stop supplementing before you test

Further testing

Physical palpation of the thyroid gland.

Full thyroid function test.

Iron (fe)

Nature of iron

Iron has a very close relationship with oxygen and energy.

With respect to emotional behaviours, iron overload appears to alter anxiety-like behaviour and mood, resulting in short tempers and anger. Too little iron, though, and you will be tired! Iron, like copper, is good when in balance, and not good at either end of being imbalanced. Iron helps us transport oxygen and gives us energy. However; it also causes oxidation (not a good thing as that is what ages us) and can be seen as red deposits on metals in everyday life, otherwise known as rust!

Dosage considerations

Optimal forms: Ferrous gluconate, fumarate, and citrate salts; combine with ascorbate (Vitamin C).

Depending on the stage of iron deficiency, 1 to 5 mg of dietary iron intake may be absorbed, the average for men being somewhat less than for women (1.0 vs. 1.4 mg/d). commonly used forms of iron supplementation are ferrous fumarate and ferrous gluconate.

Treatment regimens may use elemental iron as high as 200 mg per day for adults and 100 mg per day for children. However, in extreme cases of IDA, up to 480 mg per day has been used to achieve rapid results. IV iron can be administered in very severe cases.

Frequent monitoring of iron status should be done if this treatment is continued for several months.

Clinical indications

Fatigue, anaemia, delay in growth or cognitive development, weakness, arthralgias, organ damage

Role in the body

Oxygen Transport - iron is part of the haemoglobin molecule that carries oxygen in the blood

Cellular Energy Production - iron is required in the final steps of the production of energy from food

Removal of Harmful Free Radicals - catalase enzyme requires iron. Extracellular iron is taken up by cells and transported to the mitochondria, where it is utilised for synthesis of co-factors essential to the function of enzymes involved in oxidation-reduction reactions, DNA synthesis and repair, and a variety of other cellular processes.

Sources of iron

- Seafood - clams, oysters
- Meats - liver and kidneys, beef, reindeer meat
- Nuts/seeds - pistachios, black walnuts, sesame seeds, sunflower seeds, pumpkin seeds
- Vegetables - Irish moss, chives, parsley, soybeans
- Grains - wheat germ and bran, rice bran
- Miscellaneous - red wine, black strap molasses, sorghum syrup, bone meal, yeast

How to assess need

Hair analysis can reveal the retention of iron that can occur in a chronic bacterial infection, please assess accordingly.

Packed red blood can also be used to assess the impact of the high or low iron on the red blood cells.

Adequacy assessment through blood: Ferritin, haemoglobin, haematocrit, total iron binding capacity, transferrin saturation

Iron excess assessment through blood: Transferrin saturation

Blood markers in detail:

Mean Corpuscular Volume (MCV) is a measure of the average size of red blood cells (erythrocytes) in a blood sample. Iron plays a crucial role in MCV through its influence on red blood cell production and maturation. Here's how iron affects MCV:

Haemoglobin Synthesis: Iron is an essential component of haemoglobin, the protein within red blood cells that carries oxygen to tissues throughout the body. Adequate iron levels are necessary to produce haemoglobin. When iron is insufficient, red blood cells may not make enough of it, resulting in smaller-sized red blood cells, known as microcytic anaemia. Microcytic anaemia is associated with a decrease in MCV.

Cell Division and Maturation: Iron is involved in DNA synthesis and cell division, including the production of red blood cells. During the maturation process of red blood cells, called erythropoiesis, iron is required for proper cell growth and division. Insufficient iron can impair this process and lead to the production of smaller-sized red blood cells, contributing to a decrease in MCV.

Iron-Deficiency Anaemia: Iron deficiency is a common cause of anaemia worldwide. In iron-deficiency anaemia, the body lacks sufficient iron stores to support normal red blood cell production. As a result, the red blood cells that are produced may be smaller and have a lower haemoglobin content, leading to a decrease in MCV.

Other Factors: It's worth noting that while iron deficiency is a common cause of microcytic anaemia, other conditions or factors can also affect MCV. For example, certain inherited blood disorders like thalassaemia can result in smaller-sized red blood cells. Additionally, vitamin B12 and folate deficiencies, which are involved in red blood cell production, can lead to macrocytic anaemia, characterised by larger-sized red blood cells and an increase in MCV.

Monitoring MCV levels can provide insights into the size of red blood cells, helping in the diagnosis and management of various types of anaemia and other blood disorders.

Ferritin is a protein that serves as the primary intracellular storage form of iron in the body. During infections, ferritin levels can increase as part of the body's immune response. Here are a few reasons why ferritin levels may rise during infections:

Acute Phase Response: In response to an infection, the body initiates an acute phase response, which involves various physiological changes aimed at combating the infection. As part of this response, the liver releases certain proteins, including ferritin, into the bloodstream. The increased production of ferritin helps to sequester and store iron, limiting its availability to pathogens, as many microorganisms require iron for their growth and survival.

Inflammation: Infections trigger an inflammatory response in the body, involving the release of pro-inflammatory cytokines and other immune mediators. These cytokines can stimulate the production of ferritin. Inflammation leads to an increased demand for iron by immune cells to support their functions, and ferritin helps to regulate and supply iron as needed.

Macrophage Activation: Macrophages, a type of immune cell, play a crucial role in the immune response to infections. When activated, macrophages can produce and release ferritin as part of their defence mechanisms. Ferritin helps to store iron within macrophages, preventing its availability to pathogens.

Tissue Damage: Infections can cause tissue damage, and this damage can contribute to an increase in ferritin levels. The release of ferritin from damaged cells and tissues is part of the inflammatory response and helps to sequester iron and regulate its availability.

It's important to note that while an increase in ferritin levels can be observed during infections, it is not a specific indicator of a particular infection. Elevated ferritin levels can also be seen in other conditions, such as certain inflammatory disorders or even certain cancers. Therefore, the interpretation of ferritin levels should be done in conjunction with other clinical findings and diagnostic tests to assess the underlying cause accurately.

Low ferritin can affect many enzymes, such as the ones involved in making thyroid hormones, so if you see low ferritin, don't juts just think low iron, think about the functioning of the thyroid as well.

Iron plays a crucial role in various parameters related to iron metabolism, including Total Iron Binding Capacity (TIBC), transferrin, and transferrin saturation. Here's how iron is involved in these measures:

Total Iron Binding Capacity (TIBC): TIBC is a measure of the maximum amount of iron that can be bound to transferrin, a protein responsible for transporting iron in the bloodstream. Iron deficiency and anaemia are associated with an increase in TIBC. When iron levels are low, the body produces more transferrin to try to capture and transport more iron. Consequently, the TIBC value increases as there is more available transferrin to bind to iron.

Transferrin: Transferrin is the primary iron-transport protein in the blood. Its main function is to bind iron and deliver it to tissues throughout the body, including the bone marrow for red blood cell production. Transferrin acts as a carrier for iron, ensuring its transport to cells that require it for various biological processes. Low levels of transferrin are observed in conditions such as protein malnutrition or liver disease.

Transferrin Saturation: Transferrin saturation is a measure of the proportion of transferrin that is bound to iron. It is calculated by dividing the serum iron level by the TIBC and multiplying by 100. Transferrin saturation levels are influenced by iron levels in the body. In cases of iron deficiency, where iron stores are depleted, transferrin saturation tends to be low. Conversely, in conditions such as iron overload disorders or haemochromatosis, where there is excessive iron accumulation, transferrin saturation is high.

These measures—TIBC, transferrin, and transferrin saturation—are often used together to assess iron status and help diagnose iron-related disorders, such as iron deficiency anaemia or haemochromatosis. They provide valuable information about the body's iron-binding capacity, the availability of iron for transport, and the saturation of transferrin with iron.

Symptoms associated with deficiency

Anaemia	Hydrochloric acid deficiency
Brittle nails	Low blood pressure
Decreased resistance	Pallor
Dizziness	Weakness
Fatigue	

Symptoms associated with potential excess

Arthritis or joint pain	Iron deposits in organs
Diabetes	Liver disease or cirrhosis of the liver
Emotional problems, such as anger	Schizophrenia
High blood pressure	

If your levels are high, you can go for blood draws (therapeutic phlebotomy) to improve them. Some people may suffer from a genetic condition called haemochromatosis., Treatment of these people will involve regular blood draws. This will be done under the supervision of your healthcare provider.

Nutrient relationships

Synergistic Nutrients that will help you absorb iron include acidic foods, animal foods, vitamin C and vitamin B12.

Antagonistic Nutrients are phytates, phosphate, egg protein, manganese, zinc, nickel, chromium, copper, calcium, magnesium, cadmium, vegetarian diets

Further testing

Blood testing should be adequate but do further testing if required

Lead (Pb)

The nature of lead

Joint pain and mania! Lead causes joint pain without inflammation. It has an affinity for bones and can even be seen in X-rays, so when it is being detoxed, it goes through the joints, causing pain that can last anywhere up to 4 days. Lead also causes behavioural disorders such as phobia, depression, mania, and schizophrenia.

Role in the body

Lead has no physiological benefit and is known to be toxic.

Sources lead

The main sources of lead exposure include drinking water, food, cigarettes, industrial processes, and domestic sources. The industrial sources of lead include gasoline, house paint, plumbing pipes, lead bullets, storage batteries, pewter pitchers, toys, and taps. Lead is released into the atmosphere from industrial processes as well as from vehicle exhausts. Therefore, it may get into the soil and flow into water bodies, which can be taken up by plants, and hence, human exposure of to lead may also be through food or drinking water.

Children can also be born with elevated lead, passed through the placenta from their mothers. Diets deficient in calcium, magnesium, or iron increase lead absorption.

Common sources include:

- Ceramic glazes
- Lead water pipes
- Cigarette smoke
- Leaded gasoline
- Coloured ink or paint
- Manufacture of batteries
- Food cans soldered with lead
- Mine smelting industries
- Grecian Formula and Youth Hair (Black hair dyes)
- Pesticide residues

- Water contaminated with lead from industrial
- Lead-based paint
- Waste

How to assess body burden

Whole blood, serum, hair, urinary porphyrins can all be used to assess lead exposure and toxicity.

Blood lead testing is used to diagnose acute lead toxicity but is not accurate in detecting chronic lead toxicity. Within 30 days of exposure, most lead is removed from the blood and stored in body tissues.

Blood or urine challenge tests can detect a certain amount of lead poisoning.

Hair testing has been shown by the Environmental Protection Agency to be a good method of testing for lead poisoning. Several hair tests may be necessary before elevated lead levels are revealed.

How lead affects the body

Blood - inhibits enzymes associated with haemoglobin synthesis and increases the rate of destruction of red blood cells and the result is fatigue.

Bones - lead is incorporated into the bone in preference to calcium.

Brain - lead can cross the blood brain barrier and can inhibit copper-dependent enzymes needed for neurotransmitters (dopamine, epinephrine, norepinephrine). The result is hyperactivity.

Energy - inhibits copper and iron-dependent enzymes in the Krebs cycle required for energy production. The result is fatigue.

Kidneys - Lead can raise uric acid levels and impair kidney function. The result is oxidative damage to the body and potentially gout.

Minerals - lead displaces and can cause deficiency or bio-unavailability of calcium, zinc, manganese, copper, and iron.

Thyroid Gland - lead interferes with iodine uptake by the thyroid, and can inactivate thyroxin, the thyroid hormone.

Toxicity symptoms

Lead can have many symptoms. Toxic lead exposure, for example, may be expressed in some individuals as inflammatory disorders, in others as immune disorders, and still others as neurological disorders. The main symptoms would usually be Microcytic hypochromic anaemia, renal dysfunction, hypertension, anorexia, muscle discomfort, constipation, metallic taste, low IQ (children).

Symptoms can vary depending on the age of the person exposed.

Signs and symptoms of lead poisoning in children include:

Abdominal pain	Loss of appetite/Weight loss
Constipation	Learning difficulties
Developmental delay	Seizures
Eating things that aren't food (pica)	Sluggishness and fatigue
Hearing loss	Vomiting

Babies exposed to lead before birth might:

- Be born prematurely
- Have lower birth weight
- Have slowed growth

Although children are primarily at risk, lead poisoning is also dangerous for adults.

Signs and symptoms in adults might include:

Abdominal pain	Joint and muscle pain
Difficulties with memory or concentration	Miscarriage, stillbirth or premature birth
Headache	Mood disorders
High blood pressure	Reduced sperm count

Protective measures

Find and reduce the exposure. Increase calcium (reduces intestinal absorption), alpha lipoic acid (protection against toxicity) and iron (reduces intestinal absorption).

Support phase 2 detoxification.

Specific binders

Ca –EDTA

What does detoxing feel like

Expect joint pain (without heat). The problem is that there are 350 joints in the body and any of them can hurt when the lead leaves the bones. Other common symptoms are constipation and brain fog. These symptoms can be pretty bad and last about 4 days.

Further testing

Due to the variety of issues caused by lead, further testing would be based on the presenting case. You may want to ensure there is no iron deficiency as this can make lead toxicity worse.

Lithium (Li)

Nature of Lithium:

Nutritional Lithium is good for brain health. Nutritional lithium refers to the dietary intake of lithium, a naturally occurring mineral found in varying amounts in food and water sources. While lithium as a medication is primarily known for its therapeutic use in treating certain mental health conditions, such as bipolar disorder, there is some evidence suggesting that low-dose nutritional lithium may have mood-stabilising effects in the general population.

Dosage considerations

As a supplement, the most common form used is lithium orotate at around a 5mg dose.

As a medication for depression doses of 400-1000mg of lithium carbonate can be prescribed.

Clinical indications

Psychosis, depression, aggressive behaviour.

Role in the body

Lithium can replace sodium in the cells, and its structure resembles calcium and magnesium. It appears to have the same stabilising effect on nervous cells as calcium and magnesium.

Here are some more specific roles:

Neurotransmitter Regulation: Lithium is thought to modulate neurotransmitter systems in the brain, including serotonin, norepinephrine, and dopamine. These neurotransmitters play key roles in mood regulation, and by influencing their levels or activity, lithium may help stabilise mood. Lithium increases GABA activity and modulates the serotonin indoleamine pathway, thus impacting serotonin and melatonin and modulating circadian rhythms.

Neuro protection and Stress Response: Lithium has been found to have neuro protective properties, meaning it may protect brain cells from damage or degeneration. Additionally, it may impact the body's stress response by affecting the hypothalamic-pituitary-adrenal (HPA) axis, which is involved in the regulation of stress hormones. By modulating these systems, lithium could potentially help regulate mood and reduce the impact of stress on mental well-being.

Neuroplasticity and BDNF: Lithium has been shown to promote neuroplasticity, which refers to the brain's ability to change and adapt in response to experiences. It has also been associated with increased levels of brain-derived neurotrophic factor (BDNF), a protein involved in supporting the growth, survival, and function of neurons. Both neuroplasticity and BDNF are implicated in mood regulation, and lithium's effects on these processes may contribute to its potential mood-stabilising effects.

Inflammatory Response: Chronic inflammation has been linked to mood disorders, and there is some evidence that lithium may have anti-inflammatory effects. By modulating the inflammatory response, lithium could potentially influence mood regulation.

Functions Of Lithium

Decreases manic symptoms in manic-depressive patients

May modulate the conversion of essential fatty acids into prostaglandins

May stabilise serotonin transmission

Anti-aggressive action

Sources Of Lithium

It's important to note that the lithium content in these food sources is generally very low. The primary dietary source of lithium is typically water. However, it's also worth mentioning that lithium is mainly obtained therapeutically through prescription medications in the treatment of certain mental health conditions.

Here are some food sources that may contain trace amounts of lithium:

Drinking Water: Depending on the water source, drinking water can be a potential source of lithium. However, the lithium content in water can vary widely based on geographical location. Some studies have suggested that higher levels of lithium in drinking water may be associated with lower rates of mental health issues.

Grains and Vegetables: Whole grains and certain vegetables may contain small amounts of lithium. For example, legumes (such as lentils, chickpeas, and beans), cabbage, tomatoes, and carrots have been reported to contain trace levels of lithium. Whole grains like barley, wheat, and rice may also contain minimal amounts.

Nuts and Seeds: Some nuts and seeds may contain small amounts of lithium. Almonds, peanuts, and sunflower seeds have been reported to have trace levels of lithium.

Dairy Products: Certain dairy products may contain small amounts of lithium. Milk, cheese, and yogurt have been reported to contain trace levels of lithium.

Fish: Fish, such as salmon, tuna, and trout, have been reported to contain trace amounts of lithium.

How to assess need

In healthy individuals, RBC lithium is greater than plasma lithium, with an RBC-plasma ratio of 1:57. However, in patients being treated with very high doses of lithium, plasma levels are greater than in RBCs.

Urine has been used to establish lithium deficiency. Hair lithium levels have been shown to correlate with total body content. Numerous studies have shown that lower lithium values correlate with increased violent criminality, learning disabilities and heart disease. Students in high academic standing had greater hair lithium levels than average.

Hair analysis is an effective method of measuring lithium deficiency.

Symptoms associated with deficiency

Deficiency is associated with excessive aggressiveness, manic states, and depression.

Symptoms associated with potential excess

Disturbed mineral transport and fluid balance, nausea, vomiting, tremors, thirst, excessive urination, thyroid swelling, weight gain, drowsiness, confusion, disorientation, delirium, skin eruptions, possible kidney damage, and even seizures, coma, and death.

Chronic high doses of supplemental lithium can suppress thyroid activity.

Nutrient relationships

No significant relationships

Further testing

As needed by the presenting case.

Magnesium (Mg)

Nature of magnesium

If you burn magnesium in a laboratory, it burns bright but not for long. The same occurs in the body. It is used in many (over 350) enzyme reactions and is 'burned off really quickly, through stress, excess sugar, and simple basic body functioning. The modern diet is very low in magnesium, and it is the most commonly diagnosed nutritional deficiency. Even people who supplement, magnesium, often don't supplement at high enough doses to prevent symptoms!

Dosage considerations

Magnesium comes in many forms, the choice of which one to use, depends on the needs of the person.

Dosing to correct a deficiency, for oral magnesium is around 750 mg per day for adults; higher dosing may lead to diarrhoea if the wrong form is chosen, but if tolerated, can be used. The chloride, lactate, aspartate, glycinate and gluconate chelates of magnesium have high bioavailability, whereas the oxide, carbonate and hydroxide forms are poorly absorbed, and therefore may be used as osmotic laxatives.

IV magnesium is commonly given in much higher doses, up to 10 grams or more over 24 hours in hypomagnesaemia with intact renal function, closely monitoring serum levels.

Clinical indications

Constipation, insomnia, muscle cramping, twitching, depression, hypertension, cardiovascular disease, and diabetes.

Role in the body

Magnesium is involved (as Mg-ATP) in virtually every metabolic process occurring in the body, including active transport such as the sodium-potassium ATPase pump, and cell signalling, including cAMP in protein phosphorylation. Magnesium is also involved in multiple steps of RNA and DNA synthesis. It also plays structural roles in DNA, cell membranes and chromosomes.

Magnesium plays numerous key roles in enzymes involved in protein, carbohydrate and fatty acid metabolism. Magnesium plays a key role in more than 350 enzymes, primarily as Mg-ATP complex in energy-dependent activities.

Magnesium is a key cofactor in both methylation (especially in the role of COMT) and sulphur amino acid metabolism and is thus involved in the production of glutathione and S-adenosylmethionine. Magnesium is also required for formation of active cofactors from vitamins B1, B2, B3, B6 and pantothenic acid.

Sixty percent of tissue magnesium is in the skeleton. The rest is within the cells, where it performs all of its very essential functions. Magnesium is vital for the regulation of cell membrane permeability, muscular contraction, nerve impulse conduction, and acts as antagonism to calcium. Magnesium is also essential for energy production, and protein synthesis.

Functions Of Magnesium

Excretory - prevention of kidney stones

Digestive - laxative (in certain forms)

Nervous - maintains nerve conduction

Muscular - prevents tissue calcification, needed for muscle contraction and relaxation

Skeletal - required for bone formation

Metabolic - required for energy production, for glucose and fat metabolism, and for protein synthesis

Detoxification - required for liver activity

Sources Of Magnesium

- Nuts - almonds, brazil nuts, cashews
- Vegetables - soybeans, parsnips
- Grains - buckwheat, wheat bran, wheat germ, other grains
- Miscellaneous - chocolate, cocoa, molasses, brewer's yeast, kelp

How to assess need

Assessing magnesium status is challenging. Serum magnesium is the most commonly used specimen for magnesium measurement. However, low serum magnesium is not a sensitive test for magnesium deficiency for several reasons: Only 1% of total-body magnesium is extracellular, and it is tightly regulated by many factors, including parathyroid hormone, which normalises serum magnesium levels during low intake. Whereas a low serum magnesium level is suggestive of a deficiency, higher levels of serum magnesium correlate poorly with total-body magnesium stores.

A better index of whole-body magnesium status is the concentration of magnesium inside cells. This can be done via packed red blood cells and hair analysis

A high hair magnesium level often indicates that magnesium is being lost through the hair, resulting in deficiency symptoms such as anxiety and hyper-irritability. Elevated hair magnesium and calcium may be indicative of mobilisation of the elements from bone to replenish depleted stores in metabolically active tissues. Conversely, low hair magnesium may not be indicative of magnesium deficiency.

Only about 1% of total body magnesium is present in the liquid portion of blood, so measuring magnesium levels in RBCs provides a more accurate assessment of magnesium status. Where possible you can also test mononuclear white blood cells (MBCs).

Urine testing is used to assess nutritional intake rather than overall levels. in the presence of normal renal function, reduced urine magnesium is indicative of low magnesium intake. It should be kept in mind, however, that this test can reflect recent decrease in dietary magnesium despite normal cellular levels. This limitation can be overcome by conducting a magnesium load-retention test.

Symptoms associated with deficiency

- Anxiety
- Constipation
- Insomnia
- Irritability
- Fast heart rate
- Kidney stones
- High blood pressure
- Hyperkinetic behaviour
- Muscle cramps and spasms
- Seizures
- Tissue calcification
- Restless leg syndrome

Symptoms associated with deficiency

- Confusion
- Depression
- Diarrhoea
- Fatigue
- Low blood pressure
- Muscle weakness

Nutrient relationships

Potassium is a magnesium synergist in many enzyme systems.

Antagonists for absorption include phytates found in grains, fluoride, phosphorus and a low-protein diet.

Antagonists for utilisation include calcium. Drinking alcohol lowers magnesium levels. Modern day, junk food diets are often low in magnesium

Further testing

Several functional magnesium biomarkers have been described for assessing magnesium status, including C-reactive protein (CRP), thromboxane B2, endothelin-1 and Na/K ATPase. Although all of these are impacted by magnesium status, other factors can also impact levels, such as CRP elevation in inflammation.

TYPE	BENEFITS/USES	BIOAVALIBILITY
Citrate	Replenish low magnesium levels treat constipation	High
Malate	Chronic conditions like fibromyalgia less laxative effect than other forms	High
Oxide	Relief heartburn and constipation	Low
Chloride	Treat heartburn, constipation and low magnesium levels body detoxification	High
Lactate	People lacking on magnesium Stress and anxiety	High
Taurate	Regulate high blood sugar and high blood pressure (prevent arhythmias and protect the heart against the damage caused by heart attacks)	Medium
Sulfate	Sore muscles Stress	Low
L-threonate	Support brain and treat disorders like depression and memory loss	Medium
Glycinate	Treat depression, anxieaty and insomina Calming effect	High
Orotate	Promote heart health Energy production	Medium
Carbonate	Heartburn Upset stomach	Low

Manganese (Mn)

The nature of manganese

Manganese is called the maternal mineral because manganese-deficient animals cease to care for their young. Manganese is a trace mineral that is essential to our bodies in small amounts. Because we cannot make it, we must obtain it in food or supplements. Manganese is a coenzyme that assists many enzymes involved in breaking down carbohydrates, proteins, and cholesterol. It also assists enzymes in building bones and keeping the immune and reproductive systems running smoothly. Manganese works with vitamin K to assist in wound healing by clotting the blood.

Dosage considerations

Optimal forms include sulphate, lactate, succinate, gluconate and citrate salts.

Bioavailable forms of manganese include sulphate, lactate, succinate, gluconate and citrate. Dosing range is 5 to 13 mg/d for adults.

Clinical indications

Deficiency: increased oxidative activity

Toxicity: neurotoxicity, including Parkinsonism

Role in the body

Manganese is a cofactor for enzymes involved in metabolism of amino acids, lipids and carbohydrates.

Because of the role of manganese as a cofactor for several enzymes, low intakes might increase the risk of illness. Although it has a number of important functions in the body, the most important roles are in bone health and in energy production through glucose metabolism.

Physiological activities include immune function, regulation of blood sugar and cellular energy, reproduction, digestion, bone growth, and protection from oxidative challenge. Manganese with vitamin K supports blood clotting and haemostasis.

Functions Of Manganese

Cardiovascular - Arginine converts to either ornithine or citrulline, producing urea or nitric oxide (NO), respectively. Inhibition of arginase reduces conversion of arginine to ornithine and promotes conversion into citrulline, thereby increasing NO production (and decreasing urea production). Because manganese is the cofactor for arginase, lowered plasma manganese correlated with lower arginase activity and corresponding increased nitric oxide production

Nervous system - Manganese plays a role in balancing neurotransmitters, however, it is needed in such small amounts that most cases of Manganese affecting neurotransmitters, including dopamine (DA), glutamate, gamma aminobutyric acid (GABA), and acetylcholine (ACh) are reported through an excess not a deficiency.

Reproductive system - Manganese is essential for healthy growth (important for the foetus) and can aid in the maintenance of a healthy reproductive system. Manganese is also beneficial to thyroid health.

Endocrine system - required for normal adrenal and thyroid gland activity

Skeletal - Bones, tendons, ligaments, connective tissue. Manganese activates a wide range of enzymes, and is necessary for building healthy bones and collagen, the major component in tendons and ligaments.

Metabolic - energy production, glucose tolerance, utilisation of fats and carbohydrates. As a cofactor for several enzymes, manganese is involved in glucose, carbohydrate, and lipid metabolism, and manganese deficiency might affect carbohydrate metabolism and cause abnormalities in glucose tolerance and energy production.

Antioxidant - involved in superoxide dismutase. Manganese forms Superoxide Dismutase enzymes, which are very potent antioxidants. Superoxide dismutases are the major detoxifying enzymes of the cells and can support mitochondrial health by reducing the damage done by free radicals.

Nervous system - Manganese plays a role in balancing neurotransmitters, however, it is needed in such small amounts that most cases of Manganese affecting neurotransmitters, including dopamine (DA), glutamate, gamma aminobutyric acid (GABA), and acetylcholine (ACh) are reported through an excess not a deficiency. Change in CNS manganese tissue concentration may be accompanied by convulsions. Both high and low blood manganese has been associated with seizure disorders.

Sources Of Manganese

- Food, mining, and the fact that this metal is added to gasoline as methylcyclopentadienyl manganese tricarbonyl (MMT) and thus, gasoline fumes contain a very toxic form of manganese
- Meats - snails, egg yolk
- Nuts/seeds - sunflower, coconuts, peanuts, pecans, walnuts, chestnuts, hazelnuts, almonds, brazil nuts
- Fruits - blueberries, olives, avocados
- Vegetables - corn, corn germ, parsley, legumes
- Grains - wheat, wheat germ and bran, rice, barley, oats, buckwheat, rye
- Miscellaneous - kelp, cloves, tea

How to assess need

Red blood cell magnesium; kidney function, urinary ammonia markers, arginine/ornithine ratio.

Hair manganese is a valid indicator of toxicity in cases of manganese excess, but there is controversy over its use for deficiency states.

Symptoms associated with deficiency

Allergies	Fatigue
Bone fractures	Tinnitus
Diabetes/hypoglycaemia	Weakness (muscular)
Dizziness	Weak ligaments and tendons

Symptoms associated with potential excess

The organ most vulnerable to manganese toxicity is the brain. Manganese concentrates in areas with high iron, including the caudate-putamen, globus pallidus (GP), substantia nigra and subthalamic nuclei.

Frank manganese toxicity, "manganese madness," presents similarly to schizophrenia. Symptoms include compulsive or violent behaviour, emotional instability, hallucinations, fatigue and sexual dysfunction.

Other symptoms include: Anorexia, Ataxia, Iron deficiency, Neurological symptoms & Schizophrenia

Nutrient relationships

N-Acetyl cysteine can help form superoxide dismutase with manganese as a mitochondrial antioxidant.

Synergistic nutrients include zinc, choline, vitamin K.

Antagonistic nutrients for absorption include iron, calcium, phosphorus, and soy protein.

Antagonistic nutrients for utilisation include copper, magnesium, iron and vanadium.

Further testing

Chemically, manganese is similar to iron, so an imbalance in one may induce imbalance in the other. For example, iron deficiency may increase manganese transport, both in the gut and nervous system, creating the potential for a toxic manganese burden.

Mercury (Hg)

The nature of mercury

Mercury is a toxin that greatly affects the brain and nervous system. It is the "mad hatter" and can cause brain fog, extreme dizziness, and generally "mad" behaviour." Sir Issac Newton, the famous seventeenth century physicist, experienced a year of dark moods and marked personality change that puzzled friends and close associates. Later, analysis of archived samples of Newton's hair revealed highly elevated concentrations of mercury, which is evidence that supports the historical hypothesis that Issac Newton's "madness" was a result of his exposure to the toxic metal while he was conducting experiments to study its properties.

Role in the body

Mercury has no physiological role in the body and is considered one of the main toxins of concern in chronic health issues. In its elemental form, mercury ($Hg0$) is non-toxic. However, once chemically or enzymatically altered to the ionised, inorganic form ($Hg2+$), it becomes toxic. Thus, bioconversion of mercury to its organic alkyl forms renders some forms such as methyl mercury highly toxic with great affinity for the nervous system. Another commonly encountered organomercury compound is ethyl mercury that is released from thimerosal, a preservative in vaccines, cosmetics, tattoo inks, eye drops and contact lens solutions as well as a disinfectant (e.g. Merthiolate).

Sources Of Mercury Toxicity

Microorganisms in the in the human intestinal tract can convert non-toxic elemental mercury to inorganic $Hg2+$ and organic mercurous alkyl compounds. This is why ensuring a healthy microbiome is essential when assessing mercury.

Inorganic mercury can also be from dental amalgams.

Methylmercury is highly water soluble and readily enters aquatic food chains, accumulating at higher concentrations in the tissue as it moves up the food chain of marine organisms. This is why "fish that eats other fish" can generally contain high levels of mercury. Fish that contain high levels of mercury include shark, ray, swordfish, barramundi, gemfish, orange roughly, ling and southern bluefin tuna.

The most common sources include:
- Dental amalgam (silver fillings)
- Fish that eats other fish in the sea, such as tuna fish and swordfish
- contaminated drinking water
- Seeds and vegetables treated with mercurial fungicides
- Medications - diuretics, mercurochrome, Merthiolate, Preparation H, contact lens solution
- Occupational exposure - felt, algicides, floor waxes, adhesives, fabric softeners, manufacture of paper, production of chlorine
- Children can be born with mercury toxicity that is passed through the placenta from their mothers. Mercury can also be passed to children in breast milk.

How to assess body burden

Whole blood, erythrocyte, serum, hair, urine, urinary porphyrins.

Hair has been a frequently used specimen by the CDC and EPA for accurately assessing mercury exposure in selected populations.

2 Types of mercury are tested in blood, Methyl mercury, which is generally from food sources like contaminated fish, and Inorganic mercury, which comes from teeth fillings. Erythrocyte mercury shows a strong relationship with erythrocyte selenium, suggesting a chemical linkage between the two elements.

Urine levels are used to assess detoxification and recent exposure to mercury.

How Mercury affects health

There are three known ways by which toxic effects are produced by mercury:

(1) It reacts with sulfhydryl groups impairing the activity of enzymes.

(2) it generates protein adducts that are immunogenic, and

(3) its highly lipophilic alkyl forms alter nerve membrane function.

Autoimmune glomerulonephritis in mercury-exposed individuals has suggested an association between exposure and autoimmunity in humans.

Mercury intoxication, in turn, can produce a triad 3 of symptoms:

(1) mental changes,

(2) spontaneous tremor and deficits in psychomotor performance, and

(3) stomatitis and gingivitis.

The mental effects include erethism (excessive irritability, excitability or sensitivity to stimulation), depression, short-term memory loss, difficulty concentrating, insomnia and fatigue. Additional signs of neurotoxicity include loss of vision, hyperreflexia (skeletal muscles have an increased or overactive reflex response), sensory disturbances, impairment of speech and hearing, hyperhidrosis (excessive sweating) and muscular rigidity.

Signs and symptoms of mercury intoxication involving other organ systems include renal and gastrointestinal disturbances, pain in joints and limbs, weight loss, metallic taste in the mouth and increased susceptibility to infections

Energy - mercury compounds inhibit the enzyme ATPase, which impairs energy production in all body cells.

Nervous System - degeneration of nerve fibres occur, particularly the peripheral sensory nerve fibres. In addition to sensory nerve damage, motor conduction speed is often reduced in people with high hair mercury levels. The most common sensory effects are paraesthesia - an abnormal sensation, typically tingling or pricking ('pins and needles'), pain in the limbs, and visual and auditory disturbances. Motor disturbances result in changes in the way a person moves and walks, general sensation of weakness, falling, slurred speech, and tremor. Other symptoms are headaches, rashes, and emotional disturbances.

Risk of ADHD was found to be nearly 10 times higher when blood mercury high.

Endocrine System - mercury has been shown to concentrate in the thyroid and pituitary glands, interfering with their function. Impairment of adrenal gland activity also occurs.

Kidneys - mercury can accumulate in the kidneys, where it may cause kidney damage.

Toxicity symptoms

Mental symptoms (erethism, insomnia, fatigue, poor short-term memory), tremor, stomatitis, gingivitis, GI and renal disturbances, decreased immunity

Protective measures

Remove the source, Get the amalgams replaced with ceramic fillings, ensure this is done safely by a qualified dentist trained in the removal of mercury fillings. Reduce the amount of potentially contaminated fish.

Improve gut health.

Selenium, glutathione and vitamin C, can all protect against the oxidative damage cause by mercury.

Support phase 2 detoxification.

Specific binders

Activated charcoal, N-Acetyl cysteine and alpha lipoid acid can all have some chelating effects. DMSA, DMPS

What does detoxing feel like

Patients often report neurological flare ups that include dizziness and brain fog, but any of the symptoms caused by the toxicity can flare up for about 4 days.

Further testing

Assessing oxidative stress and the gut microbiome may be beneficial.

Molybdenum (Mo)

The nature of molybdenum

There is no real personality to molybdenum, however; the word molybdenum comes from the Greek word molybdos, meaning "lead-like."

Dosage considerations

Supplemental molybdenum is available chelated to metabolic acids such as picolinate (50 to 400 µg) and citrate. Ammonium or sodium molybdate are other commonly used forms. However, given its ready absorption, all forms are likely bioavailable.

Clinical indications

Sulphite intolerance and copper toxicity

Role in the body

Molybdenum helps the body process and eliminate toxins through the liver, as well as helping many enzymes function. It is a potent antioxidant, and it also balances copper. It supports the sulphation process, which is responsible for managing and eliminating toxins from the body. Often, if you need Molybdenum, it is because you have excess copper, so please read the copper chapter as well!

Molybdenum is required for xanthine oxidase, an enzyme involved in the formation of uric acid. Uric acid is a very potent anti anti-oxidant.

In animals, another enzyme, aldehyde oxidase, also requires molybdenum. This enzyme is involved in detoxification.

Molybdenum has been shown in animals to be involved with fat, purine, and sulphate metabolism.

It is also involved in detoxification and intimately involved in copper metabolism.

Sources of molybdenum

- Animal Products - meats - pork, lamb, beef liver
- Nuts/seeds - sunflower seeds
- Vegetables - soybeans, lima beans, lentils, peas
- Grains - buckwheat, oats, barley, wheat germ, sorghum

- Occupational sources - working around metal fumes. Molybdenum is used to make stainless steel, photographic chemicals, lubricants, pigments and reagents

How to assess need

Given the low total-body status of molybdenum, functional biomarkers may be more effective than direct measurement of molybdenum status.

You can assess molybdenum need by assessing urinary sulphate, elevated sulphite, xanthine, and hypoxanthine.

In blood, uric acid can be an indicator that you need molybdenum as it is a cofactor in the conversion of xanthine to uric acid.

Direct assessment is best done by hair analysis.

Symptoms associated with deficiency

Impaired growth

Tooth decay

Male impotence

Xanthine stones, these are rare forms of kidney stones

Symptoms of elevated copper can result from a molybdenum deficiency.

Symptoms associated with potential excess

Acute toxicity causes severe diarrhoea.

Chronic toxicity may cause gout.

Copper deficiency symptoms may also occur, including skin problems, hair loss, growth retardation, osteoporosis, thyroid abnormality, bone and joint abnormalities, and weight loss.

Nutrient relationships

Synergistic Nutrients - Molybdenum is considered to be synergistic with iron and sulphur.

Antagonistic Nutrients - Molybdenum is considered to be antagonistic to copper

Nickel (Ni)

Nature of nickel

Nickel is an incredible antioxidant and plays a vital role in protecting us against infections like H. Pylori (a bacteria linked to gastric ulcers). However; this is also one of the most allergenic metals, characterised by people feeling itchy, red & bumpy. Most often, people react to nickel contact on the skin, causing itchy rashes that, if left untreated, can leave skin discolouration.

Dosage considerations

No RDA has been established, and required amounts are likely considerably less than 500 µg/kg body weight

Clinical indications

Unknown

Role in the body

Nickel is an essential trace mineral that is found in soil, water, and foods, including almonds, dried beans, and chocolate. The body requires only trace levels of nickel, and its precise functions in the body are not well understood. However, research suggests that nickel plays a role in some chemical processes in the body, including:

Enzyme function: Nickel is a component of certain enzymes involved in chemical reactions in the body. It may also assist with iron absorption.

Hormonal regulation: Nickel may play a role in hormonal regulation in the body. Nickel can cause abnormal thyroid hormone secretion, which affects the body's growth and development and energy metabolism. And it may be related to the altered functions of the hypothalamus, pituitary, and thyroid in the hypothalamic-pituitary-thyroid axis

Red blood cell formation: Nickel is a potent stimulator of the formation of erythrocytes (red blood cells) in the haematopoietic tissue of the bone marrow.

Metabolism of Folic Acid and Vitamin B12: Nickel may play a role in the body's use of folic acid and vitamin B12, which are both necessary for healthy cell growth and development.

It's important to note that the overall absorption of dietary nickel is low, and the majority of ingested nickel exits the body in urine or stool. Nickel is not stored in most tissues or organs, with the exception of the thyroid and adrenal glands. There is no Recommended Dietary Allowance (RDA) or Adequate Intake (AI) for nickel, and research regarding the nutritional importance or biochemical function of nickel in the human body is limited. Consuming a balanced diet that includes a variety of nutrient-dense foods can help ensure adequate intake of trace minerals like nickel.

Sources Of Nickel

Nickel is used in the production of batteries, nickel-plated jewellery, machine parts, nickel plating on metallic objects, manufacture of steel, cigarette smoking, wire, electrical parts, etc. Also, it can be found in foodstuff such as imitation whip cream, unrefined grains, and cereals, commercial peanut butter, hydrogenated vegetable oils, as well as contaminated alcoholic beverages. It can also be found in soil, water, and foods, including almonds, dried beans, and chocolate.

How to assess need

The best ways to assess Nickel are through plasma, urine and faeces. Only acute exposure is revealed because of the rapidity of nickel clearance from blood.

Hair nickel has been measured for assessment of nickel status and may prove a useful biomarker for past exposure.

Symptoms associated with deficiency

Poor growth and reproduction function.

Symptoms associated with potential excess

In rare cases, a severe form of nickel allergy called systemic nickel allergy syndrome (SNAS) can cause systemic symptoms, such as headaches, fatigue, nausea, vomiting, and diarrhoea. It's important to note that symptoms of nickel allergy may take as long as 72 hours or more after exposure to appear.

Allergies

Kidney dysfunction

Low blood pressure

Malaise and fatigue

Muscle tremors, tetany, and paralysis

Nausea, vomiting

Skin problems (dermatitis)

Nutrient relationships

Nickel has been shown to work in a cooperative way with calcium, iron and zinc.

Nutritional Support: Certain nutrients, such as vitamin C, vitamin E, and selenium, can help support the body's natural detoxification processes and may aid in the removal of nickel.

Herbal Remedies: Some herbs, such as cilantro (Coriander) and chlorella, are believed to have chelating properties and may help remove heavy metals from the body.

Phosphorus (P)

The nature of Phosphorus

"Phosphorus" comes from the Greek word phosphorous, which means "bringer of light.". Phosphorus explodes on contact with air. It is extremely energetic and reactive but also burns bright and fast. Think of fireworks when you think of phosphorus!

Phosphorus regulates the normal function of nerves and muscles, including the heart, and is also a building block of our genes, as it makes up DNA, RNA, and ATP, the body's major source of energy.

Dosage considerations

Food sources are the best, ensure healthy digestion of proteins.

Clinical indications

Muscle weakness, bone pain and tingling in your arms and legs.

Roles In the Body

One of its main tasks is to serve as a building block for healthy teeth and bones. You may think that's calcium's job. But calcium needs phosphorus to make your teeth and bones strong.

Phosphorus also helps your nerves and muscles do their jobs. It's a buffer that keeps the pH level in your blood balanced. Phosphorus also helps you turn fat, carbs, and protein into energy.

Bone structure - 80-85% of phosphorus in the body is located in the bones and teeth

Energy production - (ATP - adenosine triphosphate and ADP - adenosine diphosphate)

Cell membranes - (as phospholipids)

Genetic reactions - in DNA - deoxyribonucleic acid and RNA - ribonucleic acid

Buffering agent, to maintain osmotic pressure

Functions of Phosphorus

Digestive - regulates absorption of calcium and a variety of trace elements. Phosphorus in excess has a laxative action.

Nervous - source of adenosine triphosphate (ATP) that is used for energy. It is also a component of the myelin sheath

Blood - red blood cell (RBC) metabolism

Muscular - adenosine triphosphate (ATP) needed for muscle contraction

Skeletal - Phosphorus is a major component of bone and teeth

Immune - adenosine triphosphate (ATP) for leukocytes (White blood cells).

Metabolic - energy production via phosphorylation reactions

Detoxification - adenosine triphosphate (ATP) in the liver and kidneys ensures healthy detoxification

Sources Of Phosphorus

Because phosphorus is essential to all living things, including plants and animals, it's in almost everything you eat and drink.

Manufacturers also add it to processed food

- Seafood - tuna, mackerel, pike, red snapper, salmon, sardines, whitefish, scallops, shad, smelt, anchovies, bass, bluefish, carp, caviar, eel, halibut, herring, trout
- Meats - liver (beef, chicken, hog, lamb), rabbit, sweetbreads, turkey, beef brains, chicken, eggs, egg yolk, lamb heart, kidney
- Nuts/seeds - pistachios, pumpkin, sesame, sunflower, walnuts, almonds, brazil nuts, cashews, filberts, hickory, peanuts, pecans
- Vegetables - chickpeas, garlic, lentils, popcorn, soybeans
- Dairy - cheeses
- Grains - wheat bran and germ, wild rice, buckwheat, millet, oats, oatmeal, brown rice, rice bran, rye, wheat.
- Miscellaneous - chocolate, kelp, yeast, bone meal

How to assess need

Phosphorus can be measured in blood, urine and hair

An elevated phosphorus level in a hair analysis is frequently indicative of excessive protein breakdown of body tissues. As proteins break down, phosphorus is released.

Phosphorus levels may increase temporarily as toxic metals are being eliminated during a nutrition program.

Very high phosphorus in a hair analysis (greater than 25 mg%) can indicate a serious metabolic disturbance.

A low phosphorus level is frequently associated with inadequate protein synthesis.

A low phosphorus level may be due to poor digestion or assimilation of protein. This may be due to digestive enzyme deficiency, low hydrochloric acid level, or other factors.

Although most diets are adequate in phosphorus, those on low-protein diets or vegetarians may have a low phosphorus intake.

Zinc is required for protein synthesis. Often, a low phosphorus level is associated with a zinc deficiency, cadmium toxicity, or zinc loss. When these imbalances are corrected, the phosphorus level improves.

Symptoms associated with deficiency

Poor appetite

Anaemia

Muscle weakness

Bone pain

Bone disease (osteomalacia, rickets)

Confusion

Increased susceptibility to infections

Symptoms associated with potential excess

A toxicity from phosphorus, called hyperphosphatemia, is rare because the body will regulate any excess levels in healthy individuals. It might occur with supplement use, but generally the use of phosphorus supplements is not common and the amount of phosphorus in them is typically not high.

People with hyperphosphatemia may show no symptoms; others may develop calcium deposits and hardening of soft tissues in the body, such as in the kidney, resulting from a disruption in the normal metabolism of calcium.

Nutrient relationships

Synergistic nutrients for absorption - sodium, potassium, low calcium diet, vitamin D, parathyroid hormone, high fat diet.

Metabolic utilisation- calcium, magnesium, B-complex vitamins (in energy production)

Antagonistic nutrients absorption - calcium, aluminium, iron, magnesium, vegetarian diets (specifically those high in phytates), vitamin D deficiency

Further testing

Assess calcium, PTH and vitamin D

Potassium (K)

The nature of Potassium:

Potassium keeps us energised and alive!

Dosage considerations

Citrate or chloride salts are the best forms to supplement.

Clinical indications

Hypertension, stroke, kidney stones, osteoporosis.

Enhance energy production

Prevent strokes

Treat muscle cramps

Certain medications (like diuretics) increase the need for Potassium

Role in the body

Potassium is vital for triggering the action potential for muscle and nerve cell activity.

Regulation of Thyroid Hormones: Potassium is involved in the regulation of thyroid hormones, which play a crucial role in metabolism and energy production

Fluid Balance: Potassium helps maintain normal levels of fluid inside our cells. It works in conjunction with sodium, which maintains normal fluid levels outside of cells. This balance is crucial for proper hydration and the functioning of cells.

Muscle Contraction: Potassium plays a vital role in muscle contraction, including the contraction of the heart muscle. It helps regulate the electrical impulses that allow muscles to contract and relax properly.

Nerve Function: Potassium is essential for nerve function and the transmission of nerve signals. It helps maintain the electrical potential across cell membranes, allowing nerves to send and receive signals effectively. Adequate potassium intake can help prevent nerve-related symptoms of thyroid dysfunction, such as tingling or numbness.

Blood Pressure Regulation: Potassium helps regulate blood pressure by counteracting the effects of sodium. Adequate potassium intake is associated with lower blood pressure levels and a reduced risk of hypertension.

Supports Kidney Function: Potassium plays a role in maintaining kidney health and function. It helps support proper filtration and excretion of waste products by the kidneys.

Bone Health: Some studies suggest that potassium may contribute to bone health by reducing calcium loss and promoting bone mineral density.

Functions Of Potassium

Circulatory - Through its interaction with Sodium, Potassium can lower the heart rate, dilate arteries, and can reduce blood pressure.

Excretory - A very important function of Potassium is that it maintains acid-base balance of the body.

Digestive - Potassium increases digestive tract activity.

Endocrine - Potassium helps raise aldosterone and other hormones.

Metabolic - Potassium is involved in carbohydrate metabolism.

Muscular - Potassium helps muscles to contract.

Nervous - Potassium assists with the transmitting nerve signals between organs.

Sources Of Potassium

- Seafood - Halibut, herring, lingcod, sardines
- Meats - Goose
- Nuts/seeds - Pecans, sesame, sunflower, walnuts, almonds, brazil nuts, cashews, chestnuts, filberts, peanuts
- Fruits - avocados, dates, figs, prunes, raisins
- Vegetables - Watercress, garlic, horseradish, lentils, parsley, potatoes, spinach, artichokes, lima beans, beet greens, swiss chard, collards
- Grains - Buckwheat, rye, wheat bran
- Miscellaneous - Chocolate, molasses, mushrooms, kelp, yeast, salt substitutes

How to assess need

Hair, blood, and urine can all assess potassium levels. Red blood cells may be the best specimen for assessing intracellular potassium status.

Blood is most commonly used when assessing kidney function.

Hair is useful when assessing the adrenal and thyroid function roles of potassium. Assess this with the sodium/potassium relationship and the calcium/potassium relationship.

High hair levels of potassium can indicate high sugar and glucocorticoid levels.

Very high potassium can be a potassium loss due to excessive breakdown of body cells.

Low levels in a hair analysis can indicate adrenal gland exhaustion.

Very low potassium is associated with allergies, fatigue, low blood sugar, sweet cravings, and low blood pressure

Symptoms associated with deficiency

Constipation	Muscle weakness
Fatigue	Irregular heartbeat
Low blood pressure	Skin problems
Low blood sugar (hypoglycaemia)	Water retention

Symptoms associated with potential excess

Depression

Muscle spasms

Weakness, muscle

High blood sugar (diabetes)

Nutrient relationships

Synergistic with magnesium

Antagonistic to calcium

Further testing

Assess the thyroid and adrenal glands

Selenium (Se)

The nature of Selenium

Although Selenium has no real personality, Selenium plays a crucial role in various functions in the body and is a very potent anti-oxidant.

Dosage considerations

Optimal forms include mixed selenocompounds including: selenocysteine, selenomethionine, Se-methylselenocysteine.

Clinical indications

Compromised immunity, male & female reproductive health, cardiovascular health, inflammation regulation in asthma and thyroid hormone metabolism.

Role in the body

Supplementation with selenium in patients with autoimmune thyroiditis has been shown to significantly reduce antibody production and oxidative stress. Additionally, low serum selenium is associated with increased risk of thyroid cancer.

Individuals with elevated body burden of toxic elements have greater difficulty maintaining sufficient selenium status. Selenium is able to form seleno-glutathionyl arsinium ions that are excreted in bile as well as in- soluble selenides with both arsenic, and mercury. Although the formation of such compounds reduces toxic effects of the heavy metals by sequestering them as selenocompounds, depletion of the available selenium pool could lead to selenium deficiency.

Antioxidant Activity: Selenium is a component of antioxidant enzymes, such as glutathione peroxidase, which helps protect cells from oxidative damage.

Thyroid Function: Selenium is involved in the synthesis and metabolism of thyroid hormones. It helps convert the inactive form of thyroid hormone (T4) into the active form (T3). Adequate selenium levels are important for proper thyroid function.

Immune System Support: Selenium plays a role in supporting the immune system. It helps regulate immune responses and promotes the production of antibodies.

Reproductive Health: Selenium is involved in male and female reproductive health. It is important for sperm production in men and plays a role in the development of healthy eggs in women.

Selenium helps maintain the circulatory system, digestive organs, and reproductive system. It is also involved with heavy metal detoxification.

Functions Of Selenium

Circulatory - Selenium is needed for healthy heart muscle. Low selenium levels have been linked to an increased risk of heart disease.

Excretory - Selenium increases protection from the effects of toxic metals.

Digestive - selenium may benefit gut health by reducing intestinal irritation. Intestinal irritation may be due to various factors or causes, including invading bacteria, immune system issues, or other bodily problems.

Nervous - Selenium can infer protection from the negative effects of mercury and cadmium.

Reproductive - Selenium affects uterine function and embryonic growth and gene expression. Similarly, Selenium improves testicular function including sperm count, morphology and motility, and fertility.

Endocrine - Selenium is important for thyroid and reproductive hormones.

Blood - Selenoproteins help to protect cell membranes from damage by free radicals and keep blood platelets from becoming sticky.

Skin - Selenium can help prevent skin aging. Selenium fights free radicals, minimises skin damage and inflammation, and may even prevent skin cancer. Selenium also reduces Inflammation caused by ultraviolet rays, stress, poor diet, and lack of minerals. Selenium fights inflammatory cytokines that eventually cause skin damage.

Immune - Selenium, along with other minerals, can help boost white blood cells, which improves the body's ability to fight illness and infection.

Detoxification - Selenium helps remove mercury, cadmium, silver, arsenic and peroxides.

Excess selenium intake, usually from supplements, can lead to selenium toxicity.

Sources of selenium

The amount of selenium in foods can vary widely depending on the selenium content of the soil in which it is grown. Soil content varies widely by region. Plant foods obtain selenium from soil, which will then affect the amount of selenium in animals eating those plants. Protein foods from animals are generally good sources of selenium. Seafood, organ meats, and Brazil nuts are the foods highest in selenium although Americans obtain most of their selenium from everyday staples, like breads, cereals, poultry, red meat, and eggs.

- Brazil nuts
- Fin fish and shellfish
- Beef
- Turkey
- Chicken
- Fortified cereals
- Whole-wheat bread
- Beans, lentils

How to assess need

RBC, whole blood, hair or serum selenium, plasma selenoprotein P, urinary selenosugar.

High hair selenium can be due to the use of shampoos containing selenium but may indicate a loss of selenium through the hair.

Low hair selenium may be due to dietary deficiency, which is relatively common, especially among those who eat refined foods.

It's important to note that selenium deficiency and toxicity are both relatively uncommon and can be prevented by consuming a balanced diet that includes selenium-rich foods, such as Brazil nuts, seafood, poultry, eggs, and whole grains.

Symptoms associated with deficiency

In a selenium-deficient state, oxidation of metallothionein may lead to the uncontrolled release of metals, especially copper and cadmium, thereby contributing to toxicity.

Compromised immunity	Muscle tenderness
Fatigue	Nail brittleness or discolouration
Irritability	Nausea and diarrhoea
Fatigue	Skin rash
Hair loss	Skin flushing
Metallic taste in mouth	Thyroid dysfunction

Symptoms associated with potential excess

These are very rare but can include garlic breath odour, thick brittle fingernails, dry brittle hair, red swollen skin of the hands and feet, and nervous system abnormalities including numbness, convulsions or paralysis as well as any of the following:

Altered mental states	Lethargy
Coma	Nausea and vomiting
Headaches	Seizures

Nutrient relationships

Synergistic for utilisation - vitamin C, vitamin E, glutathione.

Synergistic for absorption - amino acids, peptides, proteins.

Antagonistic for utilisation - silver, arsenic, mercury, cadmium, titanium.

Antagonistic for absorption - copper, mercury, silver, sulphate.

Sodium (Na)

The nature of sodium

Sodium is referred to as the volatility mineral and is often associated with inflammation and volatile anger.

Dosage considerations

Best sources are earth salts

Clinical indications

hypotension, tachycardia and other heart disturbances.

Role in the body

Sodium is an extracellular element involved in fluid balance, regulation of blood pressure, and cell membrane permeability.

Functions Of sodium

Circulatory - Sodium is well known in its role in the maintenance of blood pressure. It can also increase the heart rate

Excretory - Along with Potassium, Sodium helps maintain acid-base balance.

Digestive - Sodium chloride is required to produce hydrochloric acid in the stomach. When a person is under chronic stress, much of the Sodium chlorides needed for the stomach to be acidic, is excreted by the kidneys. This demonstrates one of the important links between chronic stress and poor digestion.

Endocrine -Sodium reduces aldosterone secretion.

Detoxification -Sodium keeps toxic substances in solution

Sources Of sodium

- *Table salt*
- *Seafood* - tuna, clams, caviar, lobster, sardines, scallops, shrimp
- *Meats* - brains, eggs, beef kidneys, beef liver
- *Vegetables* - beet greens, celery, Swiss chard, olives, peas
- *Dairy* - butter, buttermilk, cheeses

- *Miscellaneous* - pickles, table salt, soy sauce, steak sauce, kelp, brewer's yeast, drinking water from water softeners. Processed and fast foods are often high in salt content.

How to assess need

Sodium is assessed through blood, hair, and urine tests.

Sodium in a hair analysis is an excellent indicator of impaired adrenal gland activity.

Very low sodium is indicative of exhaustion.

A high level in a hair analysis may be indicative of excessive adrenal gland activity.

Sodium levels in a hair analysis can be elevated by toxic metals, especially cadmium.

Symptoms associated with deficiency

Allergies	Fatigue
Anorexia	Low blood pressure
Apathy	Low hydrochloric acid level
Bloating	Poor protein digestion
Depression	Slow oxidation
Dizziness	Weakness

Symptoms associated with a potential excess

Headaches	Lowers calcium and magnesium levels
High blood pressure	Nervousness
Inflammation	Oedema
Irritability	Water retention

Nutrient relationships

Synergistic nutrients include manganese, chromium, vitamin C, E and B complex.

Liquorice (the herb) can also increase sodium retention in the body.

Antagonistic nutrients include calcium, zinc, choline, inositol

Strontium (Sr)

The nature of strontium

Strontium has no known personality but has been shown to improve bone strength when supplemented.

Dosage considerations

125-680mg; A few caveats regarding strontium therapy should be considered. Strontium competes with calcium for GI absorption.

Vitamin D will initially improve strontium absorption, but high-dose strontium inhibits vitamin D formation and induces depletion of the vitamin D pool. Therefore, practitioners routinely add vitamin D and calcium. High doses or long-term therapy with strontium salts has definite risk of inducing nutrient depletions, as well as the potential for weakening the bone strength.

Clinical indications

Osteopenia, osteoporosis

Role in the body

Strontium incorporates into hydroxyl crystal lattice of bone, stimulates new cortical and cancellous bone formation, and decreases bone resorption by inhibiting osteoclastic activity (osteoclasts are the cells that break down bone). These effects are shown to occur during strontium supplementation only and decrease after the cessation of therapy.

Sources of strontium

Air and soil naturally contain small levels of non-radioactive strontium. Foods like fish, vegetables, and livestock naturally contain low levels of non-radioactive strontium. Strontium is naturally present in surface water and groundwater.

How to assess need

Serum strontium levels have been evaluated during therapy to establish absorption from the gut.

Urinary calcium and serum vitamin D can be used to monitor effects on these nutrients.

Hair strontium is commonly measured, although there is little evidence linking it to bone levels. Strontium has been shown to concentrate in hair with increased environmental exposure.

Bone resorption tests such as deoxypyridinoline, pyridinoline, bone-specific alkaline phosphatase or C-telopeptide of type I collagen may be used to establish reduction in bone resorption due to strontium therapy.

NOTE: Interpretation of DEXA results must allow for the false attenuation of strontium.

Symptoms associated with deficiency

Bone loss

Symptoms associated with potential excess

Calcium and vitamin D imbalance symptoms.

Nutrient relationships

Calcium and vitamin D

Further testing

Other assessment tools, including calcium and vitamin D assessment and bone resorption markers, should be considered

Zinc (Zn)

The nature of zinc

Zinc is the 'masculine' mineral because of its strong effect on testosterone. Its nature is protective, and this nature can be seen in the effect on the immune system. Note any white spots on nails, as this is a common sign of zinc deficiency.

Dosage considerations

It is important to dose according to gender, women tend to do well around 20mg /day and men can go to 40-50mg /day. 100mg/ day can be used for short term repletion.

Clinical indications

Depressed growth, poor immune function, alopecia, eye and skin lesions, diarrhoea. A very common indicator of zinc need are white spots on the nails.

Role in the body

Zinc is necessary for growth and development of all living organisms due to its role in numerous catalytic and regulatory enzymes and in protein folding and receptor binding. It is a cofactor for more than 300 known enzymes.

- Immune health (Zinc is a potent anti-viral)
- Activator of many key enzymes
- Growth and development
- Male reproductive system health
- Insulin production and secretion
- Prevention of the negative effects of cadmium and copper toxicity

Functions of zinc

Circulatory - Zinc maintains the health of artery walls. After a heart attack, replenishing with zinc has been shown to improve cardiac function and prevent further damage.

Respiratory - Zinc assists with the removal of carbon dioxide and maintenance of acid-base balance

Digestive - Zinc plays a vital role in the production of digestive enzymes. Zinc carnosine supports the gastrointestinal system by protecting its mucus membrane, aiding in the repair of damaged epithelial cells, inhibiting inflammation, and exhibiting antioxidant-like properties. If you take too much, or on an empty stomach, you may feel nauseous! So please only take zinc after meals.

Nervous - Zinc is one of the most abundant metal ions in the central nervous system (CNS), where it plays a crucial role in both physiological and pathological brain functions. Zinc promotes antioxidant effects, neurogenesis, and immune system responses.

Special senses - Zinc play a role in appetite regulation, as well as our sense of smell, and taste. When you lose your sense of smell and/or taste, please think of zinc.

Reproductive - Zinc plays a role in male sexual health by maintaining healthy testes and prostate. Zinc is very important in male fertility. In women it can help with oestrogen dominance and conditions such as PMS or PCOS.

Endocrine - Higher serum zinc concentrations are associated with increased insulin sensitivity. It also plays a role pituitary gonadotropin secretion, which then leads to male and female sex hormone secretion.

Blood -Zinc supplementation influences haemoglobin production.

Skeletal - Zinc can play a role in preventing osteoporosis. Zinc is an essential mineral that is required for normal skeletal growth and bone homeostasis. Furthermore, zinc appears to be able to promote bone regeneration.

Skin -Even mild deficiencies in zinc can impair collagen production, fatty acid metabolism and wound healing. Zinc is needed for building keratin and for the formation of the skin's structural protein – collagen. In fact, collagen in the skin is produced by zinc-dependent enzymes called collagenases.

Protective - Zinc's role in wound healing is multifactorial, and it is required for collagen and protein synthesis, cell proliferation, and immune function, all of which are essential for tissue regeneration and repair. All proliferating cells, including inflammatory cells, epithelial cells, and fibroblasts, require zinc.

Metabolic - Through its action on Insulin, zinc plays a role in normal carbohydrate and protein metabolism

Detoxification - Zinc assists in removing the toxic accumulation of cadmium and copper

Psychological - As it balances Copper that can contribute to mental health issues, Zinc can be used as a powerful mood stabiliser and 'sedative' mineral.

Sources of zinc

- Seafood - oysters, herring
- Meats - beef, lamb, beef, and pork liver
- Nuts/seeds - sunflower, pumpkin
- Dairy - cheese
- Grains - wheat germ
- Miscellaneous - brewer's yeast, maple syrup, bone meal, gluten, tea

How to assess need

To date, there is no generally accepted standard index for zinc status, although levels of zinc in whole blood, plasma, blood cells and urine tend to fall in severe zinc depletion. Some experts recommend using both plasma zinc and red blood cell metallothionein (MT) as an indicator of zinc status, although the MT test is not a very common one yet, with very few labs offering the test.

Zinc is most stable in a dried blood spot blood test.

Packed red blood cells can be a good way to assess a supplement program.

Urinary zinc has also been shown to be a useful bio- marker, and even to correlate with plasma zinc levels, yet it has also been shown to be a poor indicator for early stages of zinc depletion.

Hair analysis is another popular tool for assessing zinc. An elevated zinc level is commonly due to a loss of zinc from the body tissues. In these cases, zinc supplements will often be recommended.

Zinc levels may appear high to help compensate for copper toxicity. Thus, high zinc can be a tipoff of a hidden copper toxicity.

Use of "Head and Shoulders" shampoo occasionally results in an elevated zinc reading.

Cadmium or copper toxicity can cause a zinc reading to appear high in a hair analysis.

Zinc will often read low if the sodium/potassium ratio is less than 2.5:1. In this case, it is not always wise to give much zinc.

Ultimately, gathering multiple measurements of zinc status is ideal to put together the puzzle of a patient's total-body zinc status. It is also important to note that since plasma zinc is largely bound to albumin, any treatment that alters albumin levels will alter plasma zinc concentration. For example, corticosteroids, oral contraceptives and pregnancy lower plasma zinc.

Symptoms associated with deficiency

- Alcoholic cirrhosis
- Arteriosclerosis
- Cadmium toxicity
- Carbohydrate intolerance
- Copper toxicity
- Diabetes (Insulin resistance)
- Fatigue
- Failure to thrive
- Hypoglycaemia
- Impotence
- Lack of taste or smell
- Lack of appetite
- Nervousness
- Poor wound healing
- Prostate issues
- White spots on nails

Symptoms associated with potential excess

Anaemia, iron deficiency

Nausea

Depression

Vomiting

Diarrhoea

Nutrient relationships

Synergistic nutrients include magnesium, vitamin A, D, E, B6, high-protein diet

Antagonistic nutrients include copper, cadmium, iron, chromium, manganese, selenium, phytic acid, vegetarian diets, soy, cereals, fibre in diet

Novel elements

Novel elements have minimal effect but can be picked up in urine samples as they are often used in medical procedures:

Gallium

Niobium

Platinum

Rubidium

Titanium

These are considered to have low toxicity and are generally not harmful to the human body when present in normal physiological concentrations. If you have been exposed, reduce exposure, ensure a healthy gut, and support phase 2 detoxification.

Chapter 28 - Reference Section for Mould Species

Moulds can be classified as

Hazard Class A - Highly toxic mould

Hazard Class B - Allergenic mould

Hazard Class C - Opportunistic mould

Common moulds: if you see them on an environmental assessment report, you can reference them here:

If you do an environmental test and find you have a specific mould or moulds, the following is more detail on the class and potential risks associated with that mould:

Alternaria alternate –

Hazard Class B – Allergenic mould.

Alternaria is the most common form of allergenic mould in the world. It includes 50+ species. It's a velvet-textured mould with dark green or brown hairs. It is one of the most common moulds affecting children with severe allergies. Significant concentrations have been found in house dust of allergic children, supporting the hypothesis that fungal allergen exposure is an important component in the mechanism of developing asthma. Dry, windy weather spreads A. alternate spores, so symptoms get worse when these weather conditions are prevalent.

Indoors, Alternaria can be found in carpets, textiles, and on horizontal surfaces in building interiors. It is frequently found on window frames and in air conditioners. You typically find Alternaria in showers, bathtubs, and below sinks. It often signifies water damage, and it spreads quickly.

Outdoors, the fungus grows on organic debris in the soil, leaves, stems, flowers, many vegetables, cereal grains, and ornamental plants (such as cabbage and chrysanthemum)

Best test: Blood immunoglobulin test and a urine test for mycotoxins

Aspergillus fumigatus

Nicknamed "The Mummy's curse" as it may have been the reason the first archaeologists who opened the tombs in Egypt all died soon after - Hazard Class A – Toxic mould, Hazard Class B – Allergenic mould AND Hazard Class C - Opportunistic mould.

This family of fungi contains approximately 200+ recognised species. It has long flask-shaped spores that can form thick layers or walls of the mould. This creates long chains of mould growth on surfaces. Because there are so many species of Aspergillus mould, it can appear in many different colours.

Aspergillus fungi can utilise an enormous variety of organic materials for food because of their ability to produce many enzymes.

Indoors, Aspergillus can grow on just about anything given the right conditions. They like leather and cloth/fabric material a lot but are found on walls, wallpaper, PVC/paper wall covering, gypsum board, floor, carpet and mattress dust, upholstered-furniture dust, acrylic paint, UFFI, leather, HVAC insulations, filters and fans, humidifier water, shoes, leather, potted plant soil, plastic, and wood.

Outdoors Aspergillus is found in fertile soil, decaying vegetable matter, bird droppings, stored sweet potatoes, flour, tobacco, and swimming pool water. It is a major contaminant of seeds and cereals.

Some species of Aspergillus are parasitic in nature and feed on insects and animals, including humans. It depends on the species. Aspergillus species produce mycotoxins, the most well-known being the aflatoxin mycotoxin.

Aflatoxin (commonly found on peanuts, rice, and spices) - Aflatoxin is a class 1 carcinogen.

Ochratoxin (animal feed, grains, coffee, wine) – most common

Gliotoxin

Citrinin

Best tests: Blood immunoglobulin test and a urine test for mycotoxins

Aureobasidium pullulans

Hazard Class B – Allergenic mould. Currently, it is not believed that Aureobasidium produces mycotoxins.

This family contains approximately 15+ recognised species.

Aureobasidium usually grows in pink, brown, or black colour. As it ages, Aureobasidium typically turns a darker brown colour. Colonies have a slimy yeast-like appearance; spores are small and egg-shaped.

In indoor environments, it is very common to find Aureobasidium on wet wood and window frames (kitchens and bathrooms), painted surfaces that are deteriorating, in floor, carpet, and mattress dust, damp walls, and in the humidifier water.

Outdoors Aureobasidium is occasionally found on a wide range of stored foodstuffs and cereals (such as wheat, barley, and oats). It is also found in garden soil, forest soils, fresh water, aerial portions of plants, fruit, marine estuary sediments, and wood.

Sometimes Aureobasidium occurs on meat in cold stores as it can grow at very low temperatures.

It has been found in seeds, barley, oats, tomatoes, berries, citrus fruits, grapes, and pecans.

Best tests: Blood immunoglobulin test

Candida albicans

Hazard Class A, B and C *

Bloodstream and other invasive infections due to Candida species (invasive fungal diseases = IFD) are a major cause of morbidity and mortality in hospitalised adults and children in many countries worldwide.

C. albicans is what is known as a commensal pathogen, which means most of the time it doesn't harm us as it is a normal member of the gastrointestinal, oropharyngeal, and female genital flora. It is only when we become immune compromised, or our beneficial bacteria is reduced (usually from antibiotic) that Candida can become an issue. It is an opportunistic pathogen in humans as it can cause disease in immunodeficient and immunocompetent individuals that can be life-threatening

Risk factors associated with the development of invasive candidiasis include antibiotic therapy; administration of steroids, immunosuppressants, or chemotherapy; prior surgery; solid organ or haematopoietic stem cell transplants; diseases such as AIDS, leukaemia, diabetes, and lymphoma; as well as trauma and burn patients.

C. albicansis has a worldwide prevalence. It has been isolated from soil, animals, hospitals, inanimate objects, and food

Best tests: Blood immunoglobulin test, Organic acids, and a urine test for mycotoxins

Immunological reactivity to Candida (Immunodiffusion & IgG)

Stool tests (on its own or in a complete panel)

Chaetomium globosum

Hazard Class A – Toxic mould

Typically found in water-damaged buildings.

According to the Dictionary of the Fungi (10th edition, 2008), there are about 95 species in the widespread genus. Only a few species have been implicated in human disease.

Chaetomium has a cotton-like texture and usually changes colours from white to grey to brown and eventually to black over time. It has a strong smell associated with it.

Indoors, Chaetomium is found on a variety of substrates containing cellulose. It can be found on paper, drywall, carpets, baseboards, roofs, and wallpapers. Common around Stachybotrys.

Outdoors, Chaetomium is found on plant compost, straw, wood, plant debris, paper, seeds, and bird feathers.

It is not typically found in food.

Chaetomium produces two mycotoxins called:

Chaetoglobosins A and C.

Some species can also produce Sterigmatocystin as well.

Best tests: Blood immunoglobulin test and a urine test for mycotoxins

Cladosporium herbarum

Hazard Class B – Allergenic mould.

Cladosporium species produce no major mycotoxins of concern but do produce volatile organic compounds (VOCs) associated with odours. It is a major source of inhalant allergens. There are 40+ species of Cladosporium, and it is one of the most common moulds found worldwide. Cladosporium grows in both cold and hot conditions, so it's one of the most resilient kinds of mould out there. It is an olive-green or brown coloured mould with a suede-like texture.

Indoors, Cladosporium is often found growing on textiles, wood, moist windowsills, tile grout, and often in bathrooms where the relative humidity is regularly above 50%. It also can be found growing on sheetrock, subfloor, carpets, fabrics, and plywood, among other surfaces.

Outdoors, Cladosporium is often found growing in soil, on decaying plants as well as on leaves.

Best tests: Blood immunoglobulin test

Epicoccum purpurascens

Hazard B –Allergenic

This mould looks like small black pustules. It is a secondary decomposer of plants, soil, paper, and textiles. It can also be found on fruits, in polluted freshwater, on compost beds, insects, human skin, and sputum. It is known to cause leaf spots on plants. This mould is one of the more common outdoor allergens. E. purpurascens spores are more prevalent on dry, windy days.

Best tests: Blood immunoglobulin test

Fusarium proliferatum

Fusarium is both a Hazard Class A -Toxic mould and Hazard Class B – Allergenic mould, depending on the species.

Fusarium has 70+ species and, by nature, will quickly spread from room to room.

The colony texture ranges from flat to woolly or cottony. The colour of the colonies may be white, tan, salmon, cinnamon, yellow, red, violet, pink, or purple.

Fusarium are commonly isolated from carpet and mattress dust, damp walls, wallpaper, polyester polyurethane foam, humidifier pans, and areas where stagnant water occurs in HVAC systems.

It is a major pathogen of rice, sugar cane, sorghum, soybean, maize grains, asparagus, banana roots, and other fruits and vegetables.

Outdoors, Fusarium is commonly found in soil, dead or living plants, and grains.

Fusarium can produce Mycotoxins:

Trichothecenes (type B); T-2 toxin

Zearalenone

Citrinin

Best tests: Blood immunoglobulin test, Organic acids, and a urine test for mycotoxins. In the case of Fusarium. Due to the mycotoxin Zearanolone that it produces having an oestrogen effect; testing hormones is also recommended.

Mucor racemosus

Hazard Class B – Allergenic mould.

There are about 50 species of Mucor worldwide, and it requires very high levels of humidity to flourish.

Mucor usually grows in thick patches. It is often white or greyish in colour. It can also be beige or brown. It most often grows near air conditioning, HVAC systems, and ducting due to moisture from condensation. Old, damp carpets can also grow Mucor spores.

It is common on diseased pineapple, fruit juice, marmalade, and in certain soft cheeses.

Mucor is often found in soil, dead plant material, horse dung, fruits, and fruit juice. It is also found in leather, meat, dairy products, animal hair, and jute (burlap and hessian).

Best tests: Blood immunoglobulin test.

Penicillium chrysogenum

Hazard Class A – Toxic mould and B Allergenic mould.

There are 200+ species of Penicillium, and it is one of the most common moulds. It is known for its distinctive heavy, musty odour and its rapid growth rate.

Penicillium colonies are usually green, blue-green, or grey green but can be white, yellow, or pinkish. Colonies are mostly velvety to powdery in texture.

Penicillium is often found growing indoors on water-damaged building materials (chipboard/OSB, plywood, wallpaper, glue) as well as on food items (dried foods, cheeses, fruits, herbs, spices, cereals). It can also be found growing behind the paint, on fabrics, on carpets, in fiberglass insulation, and on mattresses. Penicillium loves dust.

Citrus fruits, jams, bread, apples, nuts, stuffed rubber mattresses, fabrics, stuffed furniture, leather, and house dust.

Often found growing outside in soil, decaying plant debris, compost piles, and fruit rot.

Penicillium often produces microbial volatile organic compounds (MVOCs), and some species produce mycotoxins. The Mycotoxins produced include:

Chrysogine	Isofumigaclavine A	Penicillic acid	Sterigmatocytin
Citreovirdin	Meleagrin	Penicillin	Verruculgen
Citrinin	Mycophenolic acid	Penitrem A	Viomellein
Cyclopiazonic acid	Ochratoxin A	Peptide nephrotoxin	Xanthocillin X
Decumbin	Ochratoxin	Roquefortine C & D	Xanthomegin
Griseofulvin	Patulin		

NOTE: an allergy or sensitivity to P. chrysogenum bears no relationship to an allergy or sensitivity to the antibiotic Penicillin. Also, note that not all the mycotoxins it produces can be tested for, but if you have exposure to the mould and you have the mycotoxins that can be tested for, then you probably have the rest as well.

Best tests: Blood immunoglobulin test and a urine test for mycotoxins

Phoma betae

Hazard Class A – Toxic mould and B Allergenic mould.

These colonies are often pink, purple, or greyish brown on walls and powdery or suede-like. Indoors P. betae is found on damp or humid surfaces.

Outdoors, it is found in soil, P. betae will attack damaged plants and may cause leaf blight.

It can be found in cheeses, fermented meat products, and harvested vegetables like potatoes and beets. It is considered an opportunistic pathogen in humans, primarily cutaneous (attacking the skin).

Produces Citrinin Mycotoxin as well as allergies

Best tests: Blood immunoglobulin test and a urine test for mycotoxins.

Rhizopus nigricans

Hazard Class B -Allergenic mould.

It is commonly known as the "bread" mould.

The spores are small, oval, and greyish brown. It is found on damp walls, in basements, in children's sandboxes, and on food leftovers. It is also found in nests, feathers, and droppings of wild birds.

It is closely related to the Mucor mould, and its spores are dispersed in hot, dry weather. R. nigricans is considered an occupational mould as exposure is common among workers in the fresh produce industry.

Best tests: Blood immunoglobulin test.

Setomelanomma rostrate

Hazard Class B – Allergenic

These spores are black or dark brown in colour and velvet-like in appearance. Considered seasonal, spores are released in hot, dry weather, so symptoms may get worse then.

S. rostrate is found on grasses, cereals, textiles, and in soil.

Best tests: Blood immunoglobulin test.

Stachybotrys atra

Hazard Class A – Toxic mould.

Stachybotrys is one of the most feared indoor moulds, as it is known as the nefarious "black mould." There are 15+ species, and it requires high moisture content to flourish.

Stachybotrys species have a slow to moderately rapid growth rate. Colonies are generally black but may also appear dark green, white, pink, or orange in colour.

Stachybotrys colonies have a powdery texture and are damp.

Indoors, Stachybotrys is known for growing on cellulose material such as wood, cardboard, paper, hay, or wicker.

Outdoors, Stachybotrys is often found growing on soil, decaying plant substrates, decomposing cellulose (hay, straw), leaf litter, and seeds.

Stachybotrys species produce several mycotoxins that may be deleterious to human and animal health. These mycotoxins include:

The trichothecenes

Roridan E, satratoxins F, G, and H

Verrucarin A.

Best tests: Blood immunoglobulin test, Organic acids, and a urine test for mycotoxins

Stemphylium herbarum

Hazard Class B – Allergenic mould.

These spores are fairly large, rounded, and dark brown, black, or grey in colour. This mould is common in temperate and subtropical regions.

It is found in soil, grasslands, polluted freshwater, and on leaves and the bark of trees.

As a seed-borne fungus, it is seen in barley, wheat, and tomato. S. herbarium spores are commonly released when relative humidity decreases, and light is present.

Best tests: Blood immunoglobulin test.

Trichoderma viride

Hazard Class B – Allergenic mould.

Trichoderma is very common fungi present in nearly all soils. There are five different subspecies of Trichoderma. Most trichoderma moulds are non-pathogenic, but other types produce mycotoxins. This wool-textured white mould features green patches.

Trichoderma is extremely damaging to building materials. It contains an enzyme that destroys wood and paper products as well as textiles. This leads to rot and causes these structures to crumble. A Trichoderma mould infestation must be dealt with professionally to stop the destruction of building materials and prevent further health hazards.

In an indoor environment, Trichoderma is commonly found on gypsum board and water-saturated wood, wallpaper, carpet and mattress dust, paint, and air-conditioning filters.

Outdoors, Trichoderma is a common soil, litter, and wood fungus.

Best tests: Blood immunoglobulin test and a urine test for mycotoxins

If you have tested positive for any immunological reactivity to a mould, and you have assessed your environment and treated it, there are things you need to consider moving forward to prevent the mould from growing back.

Chapter 29 - Reference Sections for The Specific Mycotoxins

if you test positive for any you can reference what to do about them here.

There are many mycotoxins, but 11 specific mycotoxins are considered the most dangerous to humans. These can be measured in urine tests. If you get a positive test, please ensure you support all six phase 2 detoxification pathways, specifically glucuronidation, glutathione, and methylation. Also, be sure to bind the toxin so that you do indeed excrete it! Note that using diffusers or smelling aroma oils such as oregano, thyme, and tea tree directly can inhibit mycotoxins, so please use those as part of your program.

Aflatoxin –

Aflatoxin M1 (AFM1) is the main metabolite of aflatoxin B1, which is a mycotoxin produced by the mould species Aspergillus. Aflatoxins are some of the most carcinogenic substances in the environment.

Aflatoxin susceptibility is dependent on multiple different factors such as age, sex, and diet.

Aflatoxin can be found in in the environment or on foods such as beans, corn, rice, tree nuts, wheat, milk, eggs, and meat.

If you breathe in spores, the mould can populate your lungs and cause severe illness.

Aflatoxin can cause liver damage, cancer, mental impairment, abdominal pain, haemorrhaging, coma, and death. Aflatoxin has been shown to inhibit leucocyte proliferation. Thus, impacting the immune system.

It is extremely toxic to the liver and can cause a rash, headache, gastrointestinal dysfunction (often extreme), lower extremity oedema, anaemia, and jaundice.

The toxicity of Aflatoxin is increased in the presence of Ochratoxin and Zearalenone.

Best binders: Bentonite, Zeolite, Charcoal, Chlorella, glucomannan

Citrinin – CTN

Citrinin is associated with poorly stored grains but can be present in water-damaged buildings. It's often found along with Ochratoxin, another kidney-toxic mycotoxin.

Dihydrocitrinone is a metabolite of Citrinin (CTN), a type B trichothecene, which is a mycotoxin that is produced by the mould species Aspergillus, Penicillium, and Monascus predominantly but is also produced by many other moulds.

CTN exposure can lead to nephropathy or severe damage to the kidneys because of its ability to increase the permeability of mitochondrial membranes in the kidneys. It has a very broad spectrum of impacts, but kidneys are the main target organs. Chief among its other negative impacts is mitochondrial dysfunction, with symptoms showing up most prominently in organ systems under high demand, such as the heart, digestion, and reproduction. Both the kidney and liver are involved in its detoxification. Citrinin can impede fertility and prevent successful pregnancy.

The three most common exposure routes are through ingestion, inhalation, and skin contact.

Multiple studies have linked CTN exposure to a suppression of the immune response.

Symptoms of Citrinin include:

Fatigue, commonly with muscle pain

Reactive blood sugar

Frequent urination and water retention

Reflux, ulcers, nausea, vomiting, diarrhoea, blood in stool

Food sensitivities

Chemical sensitivities

Heart palpitations, shortness of breath, chest pain

Menstrual changes, miscarriage, and infertility

Best binders and interventions– a blend of binders and dietary interventions including:

2 Tbsp ground organic seeds as insoluble fibre binder

Go grain-free to reduce exposure

Radishes plus vegetables/fruits in the orange-red colour band

Butyrate-rich foods - butter, cabbage, radicchio, white part of spring onion, broccoli, brussels sprouts

Green tea - particularly if skeletal muscle fatigue (Citrinin-specific effect)

Glutathione or glutathione inducers, if not tolerated - ALA, NAC, Selenium

Globe artichoke (Cynara scolymus)

Resveratrol

Melatonin

CoQ10

Chaetoglobosin A –

Chaetoglobosin A (CHA) is produced by the mould Chaetomium globosum (CG).

CG is commonly found in homes that have experienced water damage. Up to 49% of water-damaged buildings have been found to have CG.

CHA is highly toxic, even at minimal doses.

CHA disrupts cellular division and movement.

Exposure to CHA has been linked to neuronal damage, peritonitis, and cutaneous lesions.

Best binders: No specific binder – use them all.

Enniatin -

Enniatin B is a fungal metabolite of the fungus Fusarium.

This strain of fungus is one of the most common cereal contaminants.

The toxic effects of Enniatin are caused by the inhibition of the acyl-CoA

Depolarisation of mitochondria

inhibition of osteoclastic bone resorption.

Enniatin has antibiotic properties, and chronic exposure may lead to weight loss, fatigue, and liver disease. It causes dysbiosis, so please check in on the gut microbiome when you find this toxin!

Best binders: Bentonite, S.Boulardi

Gliotoxin –

Gliotoxin (GTX) is produced by the mould's Aspergillus and Candida. However, determining the Gliotoxin source can be difficult since it comes from both moulds and yeasts. Many patients who have Gliotoxin have a significant fungal yeast burden of Candida and other normally commensal yeast species.

In order to evade the body's defences, Aspergillus releases Gliotoxin to inhibit the immune system. Causes fragmentation of the DNA of the white blood cells, causing them to die or mutate

This results in the downregulation of phagocytic immune defence, which can lead to polymicrobial infections.

Gliotoxin impairs the activation of T-cells and induces apoptosis in monocytes and in monocyte-derived dendritic cells. These impairments can lead to multiple neurological syndromes.

It can be fatal in even small amounts.

Commonly seen in women with recurrent vaginitis (often when there is Candida present).

People with Gliotoxin tend to be sulphur sensitive, owing to the disulfide bond in the toxin. This is one case where even though people with Gliotoxin get depleted in them. Be very cautious in the use and timing of Zinc, Alpha-lipoic acid, N-acetyl cysteine, and Glutathione as these may actually help the toxin work better. Wait until they are on antifungal therapy so that the benefit of those nutrients goes to my patient, not the mould.

Signs and Symptoms of Gliotoxin:

- Fungal skin conditions
- Itchy skin
- Toenail fungus
- Mast cell reactions
- Bloating after eating
- Sweet cravings
- Nausea
- Constipation
- Intolerance to sulfur-containing foods
- Chemical sensitivities
- Fatigue
- Cognitive difficulties
- Headaches
- Anxiousness
- Frequent mood changes
- Despair/suicidal tendencies
- Incoordination
- Multiple sclerosis-type symptoms
- Insomnia
- Frequent infections
- Delayed wound healing

Best binders and interventions: Bentonite, NAC, S.Boulardi

Dietary interventions:

Temporary avoidance of sulphur-containing foods, such as garlic, onions, eggs, fish, and the Brassicaceae family (broccoli, kale, cauliflower, cabbage, brussels sprouts)

Bitters & Bile can help.

Bile acids have an antifungal effect on yeasts and also detox Gliotoxin by packaging it up for excretion

Things that taste bitter help to make bile and can be used before meals and/or binders to capitalise on this effect

Bitter tinctures and bitter teas can be taken with meals.

Supplements that may help:

- Molybdenum (reduces sulphur reactions)
- Antifungals as soon as possible (blends work best since this is both a yeast and mould toxin - resveratrol, antifungal bioflavonoid)
- Turmeric (antifungal detoxifying agent)
- Quercetin (reduces mast cell reactions)
- Coffee enema (induces bile secretion)
- Zinc (take with food, combats the immunotoxic effects - may cause nausea on an empty stomach, so start very low, and only once on antifungal therapy
- Glutathione* (replete deficiencies in the mitochondria. Use the same caution with thiol-containing glutathione inducers - Alpha lipoic acid (ALA), N-acetyl cysteine, and EDTA. Adding Selenomethionine helps to combat the immunotoxic effects)

*Start very low and only once on antifungal therapy

Mycophenolic acid -

Mycophenolic Acid (MPA) is produced by the Penicillium fungus.

MPA is an immunosuppressant that inhibits the proliferation of B and T lymphocytes and allows opportunistic infections to thrive

MPA exposure can increase the risk of opportunistic infections such as Clostridia and Candida. MPA is associated with miscarriage and congenital malformations when the woman is exposed in pregnancy.

It is also used as a drug in organ transplants or in autoimmune diseases, so please alert the lab if they are on immune suppressant drugs, as it will falsely elevate the results.

It is also in blue cheese – so if you or your patient eats loads of blue cheese, ask them to stop before doing the test.

Best binders – no specific binder- use them all.

Ochratoxin A –

This is a Type B Trichothecene. Ochratoxin A (OTA) is a nephrotoxic, neurotoxic, immunotoxic, and carcinogenic mycotoxin.

This chemical is produced by moulds in the Aspergillus and Penicillium families.

Exposure is primarily through inhalation in water-damaged buildings.

Exposure to OTA can also come from contaminated foods such as cereals, grape juices, dairy, spices, wine, dried vine fruit, and coffee.

OTA can lead to kidney disease and adverse neurological effects.

Studies have shown that OTA can cause significant oxidative damage to multiple brain regions and the kidneys.

Dopamine levels in the brain of mice have been shown to be decreased after exposure to OTA, this can lead to symptoms of Parkinson's disease.

Best binders – Cholestyramine/Welchol, as well as clay and charcoal binders. Glucomannan

Roridan E –

Roridin E is a macrocyclic trichothecene produced by the mould species Fusarium, Myrothecium, and Stachybotrys (i.e., black mould).

Trichothecenes are frequently found in buildings with water damage but can also be found in contaminated grain.

Trichothecenes are considered extremely toxic and have been used as biological warfare agents. Even low levels of exposure to macrocyclic trichothecenes can cause severe neurological damage, immunosuppression, endocrine disruption, cardiovascular problems, and gastrointestinal distress.

A Note on Trichothecenes:

Used in Biological warfare because they are hard to destroy and have a major impact on health including:

- Lipophilic, crosses placenta, Inhibit DNA synthesis.
- Inhibit mitochondrial function causing many issues.
- Bone marrow suppression
- Nervous system effects (pain, tremors, insomnia)
- GI distress
- Increased apoptosis
- Large vesicle on the skin (direct exposure)
- Endocrine disruption (infertility)
- Cardiovascular distress
- Immunosuppression
- Death

Best binders: Bentonite, Charcoal, Chlorella

Sterigmatocystin-

Sterigmatocystin (STG) is a mycotoxin that is closely related to aflatoxin. STG is produced from several species of mould, such as Aspergillus, Penicillium, Fusarium, Stachybotrys, Trichoderma, Chaetomium, and others.

The toxicity of STG affects the liver, kidneys, and immune system. It is carcinogenic, particularly in the cells of the GI tract and liver.

STG has been found in the dust from damp carpets. It is also a contaminant of many foods, including grains, corn, bread, cheese, spices, coffee beans, soybeans, pistachio nuts, and animal feed. In cases of lung aspergilloma, STG has been found in human tissue specimens.

Oxidative stress becomes measurably elevated during STG exposure, which causes a depletion of antioxidants such as glutathione, particularly in the liver.

Best binder and intervention – non-specific binders and glutathione

Verrucarin A

Verrucarin A (VRA) is a macrocyclic trichothecene mycotoxin produced from Stachybotrys, Fusarium, and Myrothecium. Trichothecenes are frequently found in buildings with water damage but can also be found in contaminated grain.

The primary tissues affected by VRA are gastric and intestinal mucosa, bone marrow, and spleen. VRA causes damage to human cells by inhibiting protein and DNA synthesis, disrupting mitochondrial functions, and producing oxidative stress (due to the generation of free radicals).

Exposure to VRA can cause immunological problems, vomiting, skin dermatitis, and haemorrhagic lesions.

Best binder: Any binder

Zearalenone -

Zearalenone (ZEA) is a Type B Trichothecene mycotoxin that is produced by the mould species Fusarium and has been shown to be hepatotoxic, haematotoxic, immunotoxic, and genotoxic as well as a very effective endocrine disruptor that acts like oestrogen.

ZEA is commonly found in several foods in the US, Europe, Asia, and Africa, including wheat, barley, rice, and maize.

Zearalenone is known as the oestrogenic endocrine-disrupting mycotoxin. It binds to what's considered the "bad" oestrogen receptor, which is correlated to associated risk factors for metabolic, cardiovascular, and neurological diseases, as well as osteoporosis and some oestrogenic cancers. Zearalenone is globally recognised to affect puberty in exposed children. This is not just a female issue, as Zearalenone impacts male testes and germ cells, impacting fertility in both genders. ZEA's oestrogenic activity is higher than that of other non-steroidal isoflavones (compounds that have oestrogen-like effects), such as soy and clover. Other effects that often get overlooked are Zearalenone's negative effect on heart function, the liver, and the immune system. It can slow the heart rate and decrease the contractile strength of the heart muscle. It's toxic to the liver and immune glands, which house many of our immune factories. ZEA exposure can result in thymus atrophy and alter spleen lymphocyte production, as well as impaired lymphocyte immune response, which leads to patients being susceptible to disease. Impairs fertility (transgenerational!!) and is known to cause miscarriages.

Signs and Symptoms of Zearalenone:

Hyperestrogenic syndromes	Heart block
Acne	POTS
PMS, menstrual alterations	Fainting
Precocious puberty	Dizziness/vertigo
Osteoporosis	Ear ringing
Hypoandrogenism in men	Edema
Central weight gain	Sinusitis
Infertility, both genders	Frequent infections, pneumonia
Fatigue	EBV reactivation
Short of breath, with or without chest pain	Clostridium difficele infections
Slow heart rate or palpitations	Fungal nail infections

Best binders and interventions: Bentonite, S.Boulardi, and Insoluble fibre (up to four tbsp daily)

Dietary considerations:

Kefir (protection against Zearalenone-induced oxidative damage)

Broccoli, broccoli sprouts, cauliflower, kale, brussels sprouts, cabbage, turnips)

Dandelion

Sources of ellagic acid: strawberries, raspberries, blackberries, and cranberries. Pomegranates, grapes, walnuts and pecans

Spices (ginger, cinnamon, turmeric, thyme, lemongrass and rosemary)

Ginger. Active constituent zerumbone prevents Zearalenone-induced liver injury (avoid the use of Saccharomyces yeasts, as they bioactivate)

Supplements that can help:
- Astaxanthin
- Probiotics. Lactobacillus plantarum
- DIM + Indole-3-carbinol
- Calcium-D-Glucurate
- Grape seed extract
- N-Acetyl Cysteine
- Milk thistle
- Melatonin
- Hawthorne (Crataegus oxycantha)
- Resveratrol

- Glutamine. *Not appropriate for PANDAS/PANS
- Selenium as Selenomethionine
- Vitamin E as Tocotrienols
- Lactoferrin

Laboratories that can assist you with testing:

If you struggle to find a lab that will do the testing, please go to the contact page on wwww.drshania.com and someone will be able to assist you.

Alletess - https://foodallergy.com/ - do the IGE, IGG, and IGA test called the Expanded mould panel

Analytical Research Labs (ARL) - https://arltma.com/ does hair analysis

Diagnostic solutions lab - https://www.diagnosticsolutionslab.com/ do the microbiome analysis and organic acid tests

Doctors Data Inc - https://www.doctorsdata.com/ do a number of tests, including hair analysis and hormones.

Genova - https://www.gdx.net/ and https://www.gdx.net/uk/ do a number of useful tests, including organic acids

Gut ID - https://www.gutid.com/ for microbiome assessment

Envirobiomics - https://www.envirobiomics.com/ test moulds and co-infections

KBMO - https://kbmodiagnostics.co.uk or https://kbmodiagnostics.com test for food sensitivities

Mosaic DX - https://mosaicdx.com/ do the Mycotox and Organic acids tests

Precision analytical - https://dutchtest.com/ test hormones

Real-time labs - https://realtimelab.com/ test mycotoxins and environmental toxicants

Trace Elements Inc. - https://www.traceelements.com/ and https://www.mineralcheck.com/ do hair analysis

Vibrant Wellness - https://www.vibrant-wellness.com/ toxins and gut testing

ZRT - https://www.zrtlab.com/ test blood metals as well as hormones

An excellent resource for finding a practitioner:

https://www.ifm.org/find-a-practitioner/

Visual contrast sensitivity test:

https://www.vcstest.com/

Environmental testing and rehabilitation:

Pure maintenance - they are in the UK and USA https://www.puremaintenanceuk.com/

Mould lab - https://mouldlab.co.uk/

Eurofins USA and Canada - https://www.emlab.com/

Gupta program:

https://guptaprogram.com/aff/909/

Sourcing good supplements

If you struggle to find supplements and you are in the UK, USA, EU or RSA, please go to the contact page on wwww.drshania.com and someone will be able to assist you.

I use and recommend the following brands, but there are other excellent brands that your practitioner may advise instead:

- Allergy Research
- Designs for Health
- Metagenics, Nutri advanced, Amipro
- Researched Nutritional's
- Xymogen
- Pure encapsulations
- NOW
- Dr's Best
- Microbiome Labs
- Thorne

But there are many more and you should use whatever your healthcare provider recommends.

www.ingramcontent.com/pod-product-compliance
Lightning Source LLC
Chambersburg PA
CBHW051528020426
42333CB00016B/1829